Mosby's Dissector

FOR THE Rehabilitation Professional

EXPLORING HUMAN ANATOMY

Jeff Meldrum, PhD

Associate Professor of Anatomy
and Anthropology
Department of Biological Sciences
Adjunct Associate Professor
Department of Anthropology
Department of Physical and
Occupational Therapy
Idaho State University
Pocatello, Idaho, USA

Alex Urfer, PT, PhD

Department Chair
Professor of Physical Therapy and
Physiology
Department of Physical and
Occupational Therapy
Idaho State University
Pocatello, Idaho, USA

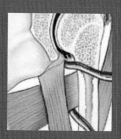

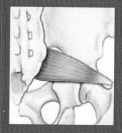

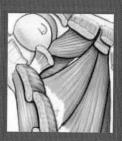

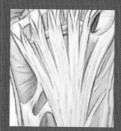

MOSBY

ELSEVIER

11830 Westline Industrial Drive
St. Louis, Missouri 63146

MOSBY'S DISSECTOR FOR THE REHABILITATION PROFESSIONAL:
EXPLORING HUMAN ANATOMY   ISBN-13: 978-0-323-05708-0

Notice

ISBN-13: 978-0-323-05708-0
ISBN-10: 0-323-05708-X

Vice President and Publisher: Linda Duncan
Executive Editor: Kathy Falk
Managing Editor: Kristin Hebberd
Developmental Editor: Sarah Vales
Publishing Services Manager: Julie Eddy
Project Manager: Marquita Parker
Designer: Amy Buxton

Working together to grow
libraries in developing countries

www.elsevier.com | www.bookaid.org | www.sabre.org

ELSEVIER | BOOK AID International | Sabre Foundation

Printed in China

Last digit is the print number: 9 8 7 6 5 4 3 2 1

To our mentors, who first pulled back the curtain on this adventure in exploration.
To our students, through whose eyes we experience the wonder anew.
Jeff Meldrum

To my students, who share the passion for learning and applying it to clinical practice.
To my parents, Adolph and Yvonne, who sacrificed much to give me the opportunity
to pursue an education in a new country.
Alex Urfer

Preface

Mosby's Dissector for the Rehabilitation Professional: Exploring Human Anatomy is a text which allows its user to move through the dissection of major body regions in a progressive fashion. The dissector is specifically tailored to the curricular needs of the rehabilitation professions including physical and occupational therapy and ancillary professions such as athletic training and applied kinesiology. The objective of the dissector is to concentrate particularly on the applied anatomy of the musculoskeletal, articular, and peripheral neurovascular systems, in contrast to the core content of medical and dental gross anatomy, which places greater emphasis on the anatomy of the head and neck, and the thoracic and abdominal viscera. The text also incorporates specific referencing to current anatomical atlases to enhance the visual presentation of their dissections. We believe that the use of the dissector in conjunction with other learning resources is an effective way to enhance student learning.

Background

This text has evolved from numerous years of experimentation in teaching and learning at the graduate level with an emphasis of uncovering what is essential knowledge of anatomy for rehabilitation clinicians. We have tried to emphasize the functional anatomy of the body wall and extremities, while also providing consideration of the applied anatomy of intracranial cavity, muscles of facial expression, temporomandibular joint, muscles of mastication, prevertebral muscles, heart, lungs, kidneys, and the pelvis. It is unique by incorporating a concise background in targeted concepts of embryogenesis, structural histology, and clinical application as recommended by standard program guidelines for the anatomy curriculum of physical and occupational therapy programs. Although focused and streamlined, it is more than simply a "cookbook" of dissection instructions. It aims to motivate the student to *explore* the human body, by posing questions rather than simply unloading

information and by pointing out the applications of their new discoveries. It encourages them to utilize their atlas more consistently and effectively as a roadmap and a study tool and bridges the gap between the classroom and the clinic via exercises and case studies that promote synthesis rather than merely rote recall.

Audience

The dissector is directed primarily to the field of physical therapy and occupational therapy (PT/OT) students, as well as other health professions students who require a strong foundation in applied regional anatomy. These are primarily graduate-level professional programs in which the students participate in a full-body cadaver dissection. It presumes a prerequisite of a systemic anatomy course or an anatomy and physiology course sequence.

Organization

The dissector begins with an introductory chapter describing the use of the dissector, including a brief historical perspective on anatomy, basic dissection technique, dissecting instruments, the importance of the clinical cases and notes, and commonly used abbreviations used in clinical documentation. Although the sequence of the 25 lab explorations is flexible, they have been ordered in such a way that the cardiopulmonary and renal organs are considered early enough that if a physiology course is taken concurrently, the student will typically have been exposed to the anatomy of these organs before addressing their physiology. All but two explorations introduce a case study to provide immediate clinical application to the anatomy which is explored. These serve to focus the students' study of applied anatomy, initiate their anticipation of clinical training, while retaining a fundamental emphasis on normal anatomy at this stage of their education. Each exploration contains explicit learning objectives and a preparation section to prepare the student for the dissection. The preparation section frequently introduces fundamental concepts of embryogenesis and structural histology that provide specific insights into the origin and nature of the adult anatomy. The lab explorations include explicit objectives, thought-provoking questions, classic memory aids, clinical notes, and employs critical figures that supplement deficiencies or simplify illustrations in the atlases. The intent is to encourage the use of and increase familiarity with the atlas, rather than provide a substitute for it. Although the dissector is primarily keyed to *Netter's* atlas, additional cross-references to the current *Grant's*, *Gray's* and *Clemente's* atlases provide flexibility in coordinating the dissector with alternate student or instructor preferences.

Finally, each exploration ends with review exercises that reinforce relationships and summarize principal anatomy. These exercises promote the synthesis and review of structure and topographic relationships, including diagramming of muscle attachments and tracing of neurovascular pathways. They are designed to effectively extend the hands-on problem-solving activities of dissection, in a fashion similar to the approach of the popular anatomy coloring books.

Key features

- This dissector is written with rehabilitation health programs in mind and contains expanded information on the musculoskeletal and nervous systems while maintaining enough core and visceral anatomy to appeal to students in physician assistant programs.
- Brief explanations of the embryogenesis and overall development of organs and regions provide an essential underpinning to the adult anatomy being presented.
- Previews of each lab exploration provide clear learning objectives and a listing of essential anatomical structures identified during the dissection of the region.
- A diversified set of case studies identifying common pathologies and disease states seen in the rehabilitation professions are presented in line with each region of dissection. A set of discussion questions after each case emphasizes the clinical applicability of the anatomy in the region being dissected. Case studies also introduce common evaluation tests incorporated in patient examination as well as intervention options to foster critical thinking.

- Clinical notes emphasize the importance of understanding the anatomy and how it may dovetail into practice.
- The dissector provides flexibility for use with several anatomical atlases which help to enhance dissections through visual cueing. Specific references to the following atlases are included throughout the text.
  - Netter FH: *Atlas of Human Anatomy*, 4th edition.
  - Agur AMR, Dalley AF: *Grant's Atlas of Anatomy*, 12th edition.
  - Drake RL, Vogl AW, Mitchell AWM, *et al.*: *Gray's Atlas of Anatomy*, 1st edition.
  - Clemente CD: *Anatomy: A Regional Atlas of the Human Body*, 5th edition.

Instructor Ancillaries

An Evolve website has been created specifically to accompany *Mosby's Dissector for the Rehabilitation Professional* and can be found by accessing the URL http://evolve.elsevier.com/Mosby/dissector/. Instructor resources are available to all adopting instructors, who can register for free access via their sales representative. Following is a summary of the resources available online:

- **Image Collection:** All the artwork from the dissection guide is available in color for download into PowerPoint or other classroom presentation formats.
- **Instructor's Manual**
  - **Sample Syllabus:** Example of how the authors teach their gross anatomy course with week-by-week breakdowns for the use of laboratory explorations throughout the semester, annotated to include objectives, sample class plans, notes and teaching tips to help incorporate this groundbreaking new guide into rehabilitation health programs.
  - **Test Bank:** 250+ questions accompanied by rationales as well as page number references to help instructors prepare exams.
  - **Additional Advanced Case Studies:** Instructors can challenge students with additional advanced case studies that offer a higher level of difficulty.

We hope you find in this text all the information and resources needed to explore the human body as a rehabilitation professional.

Jeff Meldrum
Alex Urfer

Contents

Introduction to Exploring

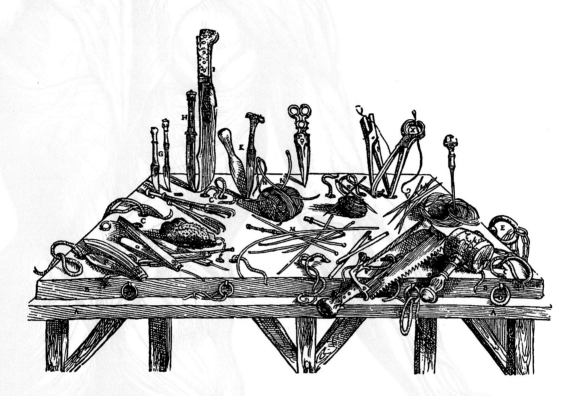

QVADRAGESIMIPRIMI CAPITIS FIGV-
rarum,eiufdemᵭ characterum Index.

FIGURE I-1
The dissection instruments employed by Vesalius to usher in the modern era of anatomy. *(From: Vesalius:* On the Fabric of the Human Body, *1543.)*

The anatomists of the Middle Ages, culminating in the works of Vesalius (1514-1564), were explorers who reformed and reestablished the first-hand study of the human body. No longer would anatomists rely by rote on the pronouncements of past authorities. Investigation was to be conducted directly and personally. This concept was the implicit message conveyed when Vesalius included a figure of his dissecting instruments in his monumental work, *On the Fabric of the Human Body*. It clearly implied that these tools were requisite to gaining, through experience, a primary understanding of the subject (Figure I-1).

With this thought in mind, we have approached the writing of *Mosby's Dissector for the Rehabilitation Professional*. To explore is to subject to a close search or examination, to scrutinize carefully. As a student of human gross anatomy, you are about to enter the ranks of the privileged few who are afforded the opportunity to explore intimately the marvelous intricacies of the human body through dissection. No substitute exists for the *cadaver experience* in providing the basis of an appreciation and comprehension of the positional relationships, topography, and textures of organs and tissues. Your *active participation* in this laboratory experience is essential to your success. Embark on this exploration with a sense of enthusiasm! Contemplate the wonder of it!

This rather singular opportunity is provided by the generous gift of some special individuals who recognized the significance of this experience in the education of an aspiring health professional. Therefore, throughout your laboratory experience, afford them the appropriate respect and consideration they deserve.

Their Bodies
By David Wagoner

That gaunt old man came first, his hair as white
As your scoured tables. Maybe you'll recollect him
By the scars of steel mill burns on the backs of his
   hands,
On the nape of his neck, on his arms and sinewy
   legs,
And her by the enduring innocence
Of her face, as open to all of you in death
As it would have been in life: She would memorize
Your names and ages and pastimes and hometowns
If she could, but she can't now, so remember her.
They believed in doctors, listened to their advice,
And followed it faithfully. You should treat them
One last time as they would have treated you.
They had been kind to others all their lives
And believed in being useful. Remember somewhere
Their son is trying hard to believe you'll learn
As much from them, as he did,
And will do your best to learn politely and truly.
The gave away the gift of those useful bodies
Against his wish (They had their own way of doing
   things).
If you are not certain which ones are theirs,
Be gentle to every body.

References

This dissection guide is intended to be used in concert with an atlas and is keyed to the figures of several of the most widely used ones, that is, Netter's, Grant's, Gray's, and Clemente's. Each resource has its respective strengths and weaknesses. The student should recognize that, occasionally, a less than point-for-point correlation exists between atlases or, for that matter, between a given atlas and the narrative of this dissection guide. Furthermore, the references to the atlases are representative rather than fully comprehensive, and the student is encouraged to *explore* their respective atlas

for all its correlated resources, just as they are encouraged to explore actively their cadaver's anatomy. Modern atlases are augmented by sectional figures, magnetic resonance imaging (MRI), computed tomography (CT), and radiographic images, which provide additional insights. A photographic atlas is an additional excellent resource but is no substitute for a primary reference atlas and should be used only as a supplement. Always have an atlas open at your table during dissection. Various computer programs and additional Web-based resources are plentiful and provide useful ancillaries for study and review but should not become distracting from the primary act of dissection in which you personally and actively explore and discover the structure of the human cadaver firsthand.

Anatomic Variation

Textbook illustrations depicting the *normal* anatomic condition represent the appearance observed in greater than 68% of cases (i.e., within one standard deviation of the range of variation). This description should not be construed as being more *correct* than the typical variations in structure observed from one individual to another. As your dissection progresses, take note of variances in your cadaver from textbook descriptions, as well as variances in alternate text descriptions or atlas depictions. Visit neighboring tables frequently, and compare the appearance of your cadaver's anatomy with that of the other cadavers in your lab. Differences in the embryonic origins of respective organ systems are correlated with the frequency of variations observed in those systems. For example, the osseoligamentous system is comparatively regular in development, whereas the vasculature is considerably variable. The musculature and associated peripheral nervous system fall somewhere intermediate between these extremes.

Instruments

The instruments employed in a modern cadaver lab are somewhat different from those recommended by Vesalius. The scalpel is essential for initiating the dissection of a new region but is frequently overused thereafter, especially by novice dissectors. A #3 scalpel handle and #10 blades are standard, but a #4 handle and #22 blades are preferred for removing large skin flaps. Do not scrimp on scalpel blades. Change them as frequently as needed. A dull blade will cost you much time and effectiveness in dissecting. A pair of small straight sharp-point scissors, in combination with a pair of forceps with straight variegated tips, will be your principal tools. Add to these implements a blunt probe (Figure I-2). Some dissections call for additional equipment, for example, osteotomes or bone saws. These tools should be supplied by your instructor.

Dissecting Technique

The first challenge encountered will be the reflection (or peeling back of) and, if so instructed, the removal of the skin. The thickness of the skin and subcutaneous fat, or superficial fascia, varies considerably among regions of the body. Adjust the depth of your cuts accordingly. Typically a midline incision is followed by several transverse incisions. The locations of these incisions are largely a matter of convenience, although specific placement of cuts may be indicated in sensitive areas. The trick is to begin your reflection at the corners created by the intersection of the midline and transverse incisions. Once a corner is reflected, make a stab incision a little larger than a buttonhole, which will permit you to place your index finger through it (Figure I-3). Place considerable traction on the skin flap, and you will see the white connective tissue fibers that anchor the superficial fascia to the deep fascia (epimysium). Draw the scalpel blade lightly across the fibers, keeping the blade parallel to the plane of

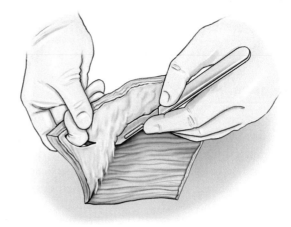

FIGURE I-3
A stab incision allows traction to be applied to the skin flap during reflection. The scalpel blade should be held parallel to the exposed surface of the deep fascia.

separation. Carefully follow this fascial plane without cutting into deeper structures.

Once the skin flaps have been reflected or removed, use the scalpel judiciously. Most of the subsequent dissection will be carried out using your fingertip or a blunt probe or by employing the *scissor technique*. The scissor technique may feel awkward at first but, with a little practice, will become second nature and will serve you well for locating and isolating structures of interest. The scissors are held inverted, the point pierces the fascia or is insinuated between two structures, and then the blades are spread open (Figure I-4).

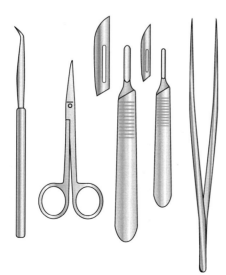

FIGURE I-2
Principle tools of dissection.

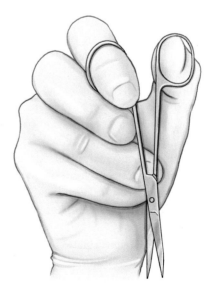

FIGURE I-4
Illustration of the manner in which the instrument is held in the scissor technique.

However, if used indiscriminately, this method can render the fascia into a clump of confused strands.

Embryology and Histology

An understanding of the origin and architecture of the tissues of the body requires a brief introduction to human embryology and histology. The derivation and fates of the three principal germ layers of the trilaminar embryo are established and discussed throughout the text. In a similar fashion the structural histology of selected tissues are considered to establish the basis for their varying textures and mechanical properties. These insights will form the basis for eventual consideration of the pathologic condition and injury of tissues.

Clinical Case Studies and Clinical Notes

Human anatomy and its progressive exploration through cadaver dissection are the major underpinnings for the study of clinical health professions and are essential to understanding the process of general medicine and, more specifically, rehabilitation medicine. The majority of the health professions are moving toward graduate-level preparation, as is evidenced by the evolution of the Doctor of Physical Therapy, Doctor of Occupational Therapy, Master of Speech Therapy, Nurse Practitioner, and Physician Assistant Master's degrees. The move toward these advanced levels of training, coupled with the *direct-access* scope of practice, have mandated a more focused approach in understanding human anatomy. To this end, clinical cases introduce selected laboratory experiences in the text, focusing the students on the primary anatomy affected by various types of pathologic conditions encountered in the scope of common general medical and rehabilitative practice. Students are introduced to and begin to engage in medical terminology, problem solving, diagnostic strategies, critical thinking, and overall patient treatment through the direct application of anatomy to clinical cases.

Each case will present a patient history in line with current medical terminology and traditional etiologic factors related to the type of condition or disease. The student will be directed to concentrate on various tissues during the dissection and to predict the possible site of tissue damage or appreciate the anatomy in light of the type of case presented. The presentation of the case will also probe student background knowledge of basic anatomy and physiology as they relate to the system in question. A major focus will be toward identifying the problem *zone* of the anatomy and why a higher potential exists for injury or disease. In addition to the clinical cases, clinical notes are dispersed in the text to highlight the importance of the structures as they relate to clinical practice. The dissection guide contains a detailed glossary of abbreviations to *initiate* the student in the use of clinical and related medical terminology. In addition, selected radiographic, MRI, and graphic images are provided to guide the student to an appreciation of the pathologic condition described.

Abbreviation List

The following list contains abbreviations that may be used for clinical documentation.

A	assessment or assistance
ā	before
AAROM	active assistive range of motion
ac	before meals
AC joints	acromioclavicular joints
ACTH	adrenocorticotrophic hormone
ad lib	at discretion
ADL	activities of daily living
adm	admission
AE	above elbow
AFO	ankle foot orthosis
AIIS	anterior-inferior iliac spine
AJ	ankle jerk
AK, A/K	above knee
Am	morning
AMA	against medical advice
AP, A/P	anterior-posterior
AROM	active range of motion
ASA	aspirin
ASAP	as soon as possible
ASHD	arteriosclerotic heart disease
ASIS	anterior-superior iliac spine
assist	assistance
B/B	bowel/bladder
B/S	bedside
BE	below elbow
bid	twice a day
bilat, B, (B)	bilateral

BK, B/K	below knee		**ESTR**	electrical stimulation for tissue repair
BM	bowel movement		**F**	fair (muscle strength, balance)
BMI	body mass index		**FBS**	fasting blood sugar
BP	blood pressure		**FH**	family history
bpm	beats per minute		**ft.**	foot, feet (the measurement)
BRP	bathroom privileges		**FUO**	fever, unknown origin
BUN	blood urea nitrogen (blood test)		**FWB**	full weight bearing
c	with		**Fx**	fracture
C	centigrade		**G**	good (muscle strength, balance)
C & S	culture and sensitivity		**GB**	gallbladder
CA	carcinoma, cancer		**GI**	gastrointestinal
CABG	coronary artery bypass graft		**gm**	gram
CAD	coronary artery disease		**GYN**	gynecology
cal	calories		**h, hr.**	hour
CBC	complete blood count		**H & H, H/H**	hematocrit and hemoglobin
CBS	chronic brain syndrome		**H & P**	history and physical
cc	cubic centimeter		**HA, H/A**	headache
CC, C/C	chief complaint		**Hb, Hgb**	hemoglobin
CG	contact guard		**HCVD**	hypertensive cardiovascular disease
CHF	congestive heart failure		**HEENT**	head, ear, eyes, nose, throat
cm	centimeter		**HNP**	herniated nucleus pulposus
CNS	central nervous system		**HOB**	head of bead
c/o	complains of		**HPI**	history of present illness/injury
COLD	chronic obstructive lung disease		**HR**	heart rate
cont.	continue		**hs**	at bedtime
COPD	chronic obstructive pulmonary disease		**Ht**	hematocrit
COTA	certified occupational therapy assistant		**ht.**	height
CP	cerebral palsy		**HTN**	hypertension
CPR	cardiopulmonary resuscitation		**Hx, hx**	history
CSR	cough/sneeze reflex		**I & O**	intake and output
CSF	cerebral spinal fluid		**IADL**	instrumental activities of daily living
Ct.	client		**ICU**	intensive care unit
CV	cardiovascular		**IM**	intramuscular
CVA	cerebrovascular accident		**imp.**	impression
CWI	crutch walking instructions		**in.**	inches
Cysto	cystoscopic examination		**IV**	intravenous
D/C	discontinued or discharged		**kcal**	kilocalories
dept.	department		**kg**	kilogram
DIP	distal interphalangeal joint		**KJ**	knee jerk
DM	diabetes mellitus		**KUB**	kidney, ureter, bladder
DO	doctor of osteopathy		**L**	liter
DTR	deep-tendon reflex		**L., (L), L**	left
Dx	diagnosis		**lb.**	pound
ECF	extended care facility		**LBP**	low back pain
ECG, EKG	electrocardiogram		**LE**	lower extremity
EEG	electroencephalogram		**LOB**	loss of balance
EENT	ear, eyes, nose, throat		**LOC**	loss of consciousness
EMG	electromyogram		**LP**	lumbar puncture
ER	emergency room			

m	meter
max	maximum assistance
MD	medical doctor, doctor of medicine
MED	minimal erythemal dose
meds.	medications
MFT	muscle function test
mg	milligram
MI	myocardial infarction
min A	minimum assistance
min.	minutes
ml	milliliter
mm	millimeter
mo.	month
mod A	moderate assistance
MP, MCP	metacarpophalangeal
MS	multiple sclerosis
MTP	metatarsophalangeal
MVA	motor vehicle accident
N	normal (muscle strength)
NDT	neurodevelopmental treatment
neg, (–), –	negative
N.H.	nursing home
NMES	neuromuscular electrical stimulation
noc	night, at night
NPO	nothing by mouth
NSR	normal sinus rhythm
NWB	non weight bearing
O:	objective
OB	obstetrics
OBS	organic brain syndrome
od	once daily
O.P.	outpatient
O.R.	operating room
ORIF	open reduction, internal fixation
OT	occupational therapist, occupational therapy
OTA	occupational therapist assistant
oz.	ounce
P	poor (muscle strength, balance)
p	after
P:	plan (treatment plan)
P.A.	physician's assistant
PA, P/A	posterior-anterior
para	paraplegia
pc	after meals
per	by or through
per os, p.o.	by mouth
PERRLA	pupils, equal, round, reactive to light and accommodations
PH, PMH	past history, past medical history
PLF	prior level of function
PNF	proprioceptive neuromuscular facilitation
PNI	peripheral nerve injury
POMR	problem-oriented medical record
Pos, +, (+)	positive
poss	possible
postop	after surgery (operation)
PRE	progressive resistive exercise
preop	before surgery (operation)
prn	whenever necessary
PROM	passive range of motion
PSIS	posterior superior iliac spine
PT	physical therapy, physical therapist
Pt., pt.	patient
PTA	physical therapist assistant
pta	prior to admission
PTB	patellar tendon bearing
PWB	partial weight bearing
P.Y.S.	pack year smoker
q	every
qd	every day
qh	every hour
qid	four times a day
qn	every night
qt.	quart
R, (R), R.	right
RA	rheumatoid arthritis
RBC	red blood cell count
R.D.	registered dietician
re:	regarding
Res.	resident
resp	respiratory, respiration
RN	registered nurse
RO, R/O	rule out
ROM	range of motion
ROS	review of systems
RR	respiratory rate
R.T.	respiratory therapist
RROM	resistive range of motion
Rx	treatment, prescription, therapy
s	without
S	supervised
SACH	solid ankle cushion heel
SBA	stand by assistance
SC joint	sternoclavicular joint
sec.	seconds
SED	suberythemal dose

sig	directions for use, give as follows, let it be labeled	**v/cues**	verbal cues
SI(J)	sacroiliac (joint)	**w/c**	wheelchair
SLE	systemic lupus erythematosus	**W/cm²**	watts per square centimeter
SLR	straight leg raise	**WBAT**	weight bearing as tolerated
SNF	skilled nursing facility	**WBC**	white blood cell count
SOAP	subjective, objective, assessment, plan	**wk.**	week
SOB	shortness of breath	**WNL**	within normal limits
SP, s/p	status post	**wt.**	weight
spec	specimen	**x**	number of times performed
stat.	immediately, at once	**x′**	x feet or minutes
Sx	symptoms	**x″**	x inches or seconds
T	trace (muscle strength)	**yd.**	yard
tab	tablet	**y/o**	years old
TB	tuberculosis	**yr.**	year
tbsp.	tablespoon	♂	male
TDWB	touch down weight bearing	♀	female
TENS, TNS	transcutaneous electrical nerve simulator	**#, lbs.**	number (#1 = number 1), pounds (#5 wt. = 5-pound weight)
t/f	transfer	**Δ**	change
THR	total hip replacement	**/**	per
TIA	transient ischemic attack	**%**	percent
tid	three times daily	**+, (+), pos**	plus, positive
TKR	total knee replacement	**+, &, et.**	and
TMJD	temporomandibular joint disorder	**−, (−)**	minus, negative
TNR	tonic neck reflex	**//, // bars**	parallel or parallel bars
t.o.	telephone order	**@**	at
TPR	temperature, pulse, and respiration	$\sim, \approx, \equiv$	approximately
		+2, × 2	assistance (assistance of two people given; also written "assistance of 2," "assist of 2")
tsp.	teaspoon		
TTWB	toe touch weight bearing	**<**	less than
TUR	transurethral resection	**=**	equal
Tx	traction, treatment	**>**	greater than
UA	urine analysis	**↑**	up, upward, increase
UE	upper extremity	**→**	to, progressing forward, approaching
UMN	upper motor neuron		
URI	upper respiratory infection	**↓**	down, downward, decrease
US	ultrasound	**↔**	to and from
UTI	urinary tract infection	**1°**	primary
UV	ultraviolet	**2°**	secondary, secondary to

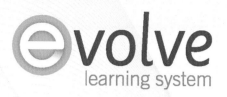 learning system

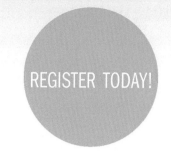

To access the free Evolve Resources, visit:

http://evolve.elsevier.com/Mosby/dissector/

Evolve Instructor Resources for Mosby's Dissector for the Rehabilitation Professional offers the following features:

- **Instructor's Manual**
  - Syllabus
  - Test bank

- **Image Collection**

- **Advanced Case Studies**

Please contact your Elsevier sales representative for access to these free resources

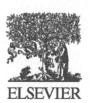

Vertebral Column

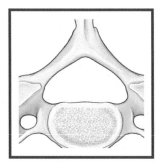

LAB OBJECTIVES

This lab is a dry lab involving the examination of the skeletal elements of the vertebral column, or spine, and their relationships to one another. On completion the student should be able to:

- Discuss the development of the somites and notocord and their contribution to the formation of the vertebrae and intervertebral discs.
- Describe the segmental organization of the spinal nerves, and define a dermatome.
- Describe the anatomy of the intervertebral disc and the consequences of disc herniation.
- Name the parts of a typical vertebra, and describe the regional homologies and specializations of the vertebral column, especially the intervertebral articulations.
- Identify the primary and secondary curvatures of the vertebral column, and identify excessive curvatures of the spine.

CASE STUDY

The Crooked Spine

A therapist is taking part in a school musculoskeletal screening clinic and is examining the students in the seventh grade. A 14 **y/o** explains that she has an abnormal gait, and she states that she appears "uneven" when she stands in front of a mirror. You analyze her posture via a grid method and notice that the **R** shoulder is slightly lower than the **L** and the **R** iliac crest is higher on the **R** compared with the **L.** Furthermore, the spine in the thoracic region deviates to the left, and the associated scapula is prominent when she is in a standing position (Figure 1-1).

On observational gait analysis **(OGA)**, you notice a clear deviation as she *vaults* (plantar flexes the right foot) as the left foot swings through. You ask her to bend forward at the waist, and a noticeable thoracic vertebral column deviation on the left is seen, which resembles a *hump*. The rest of her history is unremarkable.

Identification of the Anatomy

The forces on the vertebral column during adolescent maturation are dramatic and may alter the normal functional curves as the individual vertebral segments are progressing toward bony ossification. The vertebral anatomy indicates variations in the vertebral bodies and the intervertebral discs **(IVDs)**. The structure of the discs and bodies provide for motion in all planes and are affected by external and internal forces alike. Young children are especially vulnerable to certain forces as the spine matures.

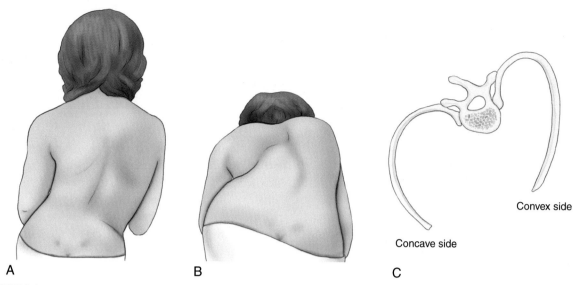

Convex side

Concave side

A   B   C

FIGURE 1-1

A, Patient with scoliosis exhibiting lateral deviation of the spine and prominence of the associated scapula. **B,** Convexity of the right rib cage produces a *hump* when the patient bends forward. **C,** The skeletal correlates of the asymmetry of the thorax.

Appreciate the following structures

Bony:

    Regional characteristics of the vertebral bodies and associated discs

    Articular facets

Abnormalities:

    Prefixation and postfixation

    Sacralization

    Lumbarization

    Hemivertebrae

    Spina bifida

Questions

1. What is this condition?
2. What is the underlying cause of the abnormal *hump* and scapula prominence in this patient?
3. What is the relationship of the gait abnormality to the pathologic condition of the spine?

Discussion

The alteration of spine curvatures in the coronal plane is called **scoliosis** and is classified by the underlying cause. In this particular case, the patient has **idiopathic adolescent scoliosis** because she is 14 years of age and has no other marked medical history related to this deformity. Other causes are related to congenital abnormalities, neuromuscular (myopathy and neuropathy), osteochondrodystrophy, and other connective tissue disorders.

The majority of scoliosis is idiopathic in nature and has both planar and rotatory deformities in the vertebral body segments. Even though early detection helps in managing the problem, scoliotic curves that advance beyond 50 degrees of deviation usually need surgical intervention. Although very rare, severe scoliosis in adults may compromise cardiac and respiratory function. Curves are generally found in the thoracic and lumbar areas secondary to the load-bearing aspects. The rib hump and scapular prominence in the *Adams forward bending test* reflect the inappropriate biomechanics of a scoliotic spine.

Normally, each region of the spine has a distinct **coupling** movement. Coupling is described as one motion causing another motion at the same time. As the thoracic spine side-bends, the individual vertebrae rotate to the same side as a function of the orientation of the **zygapophyseal joint** facets. In a scoliotic spine the opposite occurs, which moves the ribs posteriorly on the convexity of the curve, causing a noticeable hump. The scapula follows the roundedness of the thoracic cage and is viewed more prominently in the posterior position. Coupling is important in all normal motions of the spine and can be problematic in normal function if an abnormality exists.

Preparation

You will not begin cadaver dissection during this lab exploration, but you will examine and review the anatomic features of the articulated and disarticulated skeleton, especially those of the vertebral column. A preview of and continual reference to the skeleton should always be an integral part of your study of the human cadaver. Reference should be made to the skeleton so as to identify the surface anatomy of palpable bony landmarks before initiating skin incisions. Cadaver tissues are fixed and hardened by the embalming process, making palpation less similar to palpating a living patient. Attempt to identify bony landmarks on yourself or on a lab partner, or both. These bony landmarks will also be important during patient examination and assessment in the clinical setting. Also, refer to the skeleton when determining muscle attachments and joint morphology and function.

Anatomic Overview

The developing embryo begins to display a segmental organization as the **paraxial mesoderm** divides into **somites.** The formation of the vertebral column reflects this segmental organization and, in turn, imposes it on the spinal cord, with subsequent outgrowth of spinal nerves. To appreciate this segmentation better, we will review the formation of the trilaminar embryo and differentiation of the paraxial mesoderm.

FORMATION OF THE TRILAMINAR EMBRYO

Fertilization produces a **zygote** with the diploid number of chromosomes. After three to four mitotic divisions a **morula** (L. for *mulberry*) is formed. Next a fluid-filled cavity, the **blastocoele,** develops within the mass of cells as they segregate into two populations: an inner cell mass, the **embryoblast** that will give rise to the embryo proper, and the **trophoblast** that will develop into the placenta and associated membranes (Figure 1-2).

During the second week a second cavity, the **amniotic cavity,** forms and the inner cell mass becomes a bilaminar **embryonic disc.** The two layers are the **epiblast** and the **hypoblast** *(Remember: second week = two cavities and two layers).*

The third week is characterized by the formation of the **primitive streak,** a thickened linear layer of epiblast, and the establishment of the **trilaminar embryo.** Cells of the epiblast migrate through the primitive streak and insinuate between the epiblast and the hypoblast to form the **intraembryonic mesoderm.** This process is referred to as **gastrulation.** Once completed, the resulting three layers are known as **ectoderm, mesoderm** and **endoderm.** *(Remember: third week = three layers).* From these three layers, all tissues of the body are derived (Figure 1-3).

SEGMENTAL ORGANIZATION OF THE TRUNK

The mesoderm situated cranial to the primitive streak differentiates into a rodlike structure known as the **notocord.** The notocord induces changes in the overlying ectoderm, initiating the formation of the **neural tube.** The notocord also induces mesoderm on each side of the notocord and neural tube to proliferate, forming longitudinal columns of cells called the **paraxial mesoderm,** which, in turn, begin to segregate serially into clumps of cells called **somites.** This process begins in what will become the cervical region and progresses both cranially and caudally until 42 to 44 somites are produced.

Each somite differentiates and divides into a **sclerotome** and a **dermomyotome.** The sclerotome cells stream toward and condense around the notochord and neural tube. Each dermomyotome has an individual segmental spinal nerve associated with it. To allow the egress of the spinal nerve from the developing spinal canal, the sclerotomes split, and the caudal portion of one joins the cranial portion of the subsequent sclerotome. The portion that condenses around the notocord forms the rudiments of the **vertebral body,** and that portion around the neural tube forms the rudiments of the **vertebral (or neural) arch.** Thus the vertebral rudiments actually lie *intersegmentally* relative to the somites. Given that the ribs are also outgrowths of the vertebrae, they too are intersegmental.

Each segmental dermomyotome has an individual segmental **spinal nerve** associated with it that innervates the derived skeletal muscle and overlying skin. The area of skin innervated by a single spinal nerve is called a **dermatome (NI64; G4.52; GY16; C7, 404).** In reality, considerable overlap of adjacent dermatomes exists, and individual variation in pattern may be present. *What implication does this overlap have for sensory deficits?* A general understanding and familiarity with the pattern of dermatome distribution is essential for localizing a spinal cord lesion **(G4.53).** *Note the numbering convention for spinal nerves. Why do eight cervical*

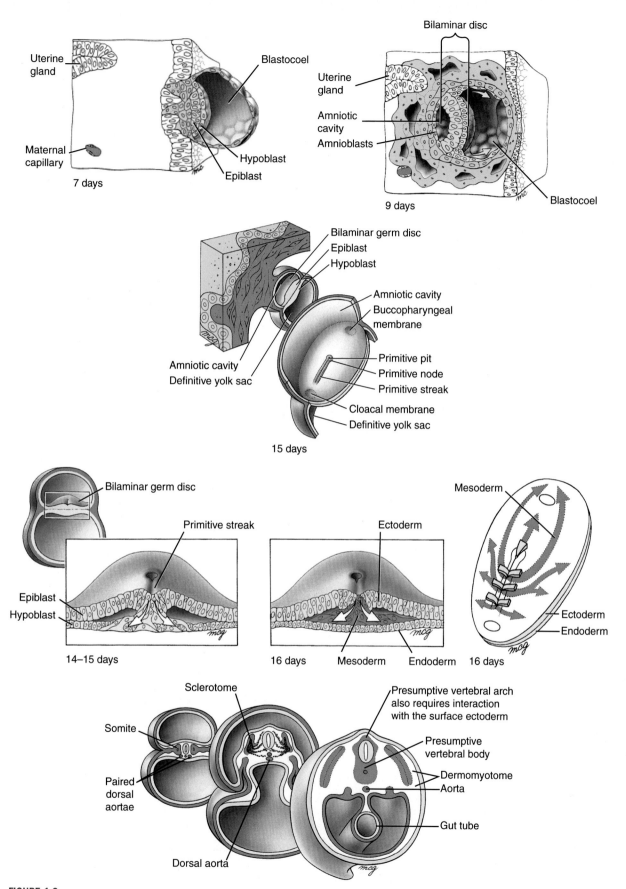

FIGURE 1-2

Differentiation of the embryoblast into a bilaminar embryonic disc, followed by the differentiation of mesoderm and formation of the germ layers of the tri-laminar embryo. *(From Larsen W: Human embryology, ed 3, Philadelphia, 2001, Churchill Livingstone.)*

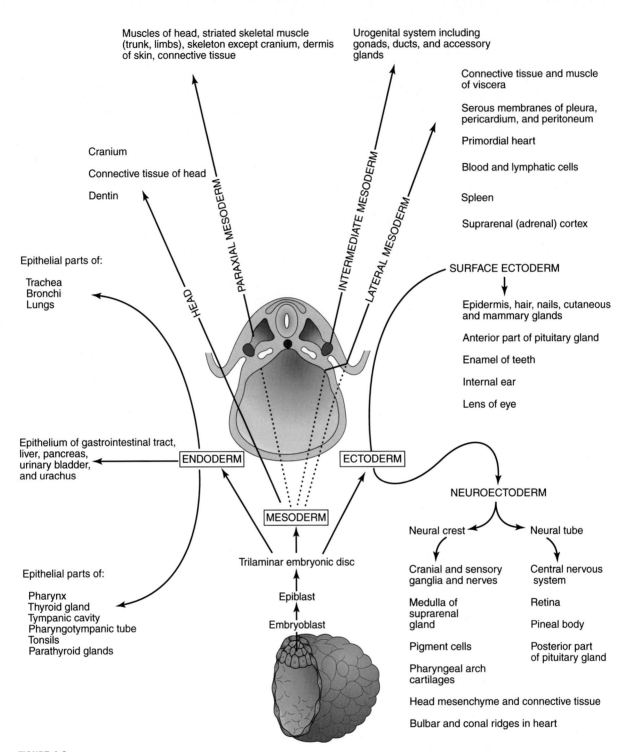

Muscles of head, striated skeletal muscle (trunk, limbs), skeleton except cranium, dermis of skin, connective tissue

Urogenital system including gonads, ducts, and accessory glands

Connective tissue and muscle of viscera

Serous membranes of pleura, pericardium, and peritoneum

Primordial heart

Blood and lymphatic cells

Spleen

Suprarenal (adrenal) cortex

Cranium

Connective tissue of head

Dentin

Epithelial parts of:

Trachea
Bronchi
Lungs

PARAXIAL MESODERM

HEAD

INTERMEDIATE MESODERM

LATERAL MESODERM

SURFACE ECTODERM

Epidermis, hair, nails, cutaneous and mammary glands

Anterior part of pituitary gland

Enamel of teeth

Internal ear

Lens of eye

ENDODERM

Epithelium of gastrointestinal tract, liver, pancreas, urinary bladder, and urachus

ECTODERM

NEUROECTODERM

MESODERM

Trilaminar embryonic disc

Epiblast

Embryoblast

Neural crest

Neural tube

Cranial and sensory ganglia and nerves

Central nervous system

Medulla of suprarenal gland

Retina

Pigment cells

Pineal body

Posterior part of pituitary gland

Pharyngeal arch cartilages

Head mesenchyme and connective tissue

Bulbar and conal ridges in heart

Epithelial parts of:

Pharynx
Thyroid gland
Tympanic cavity
Pharyngotympanic tube
Tonsils
Parathyroid glands

FIGURE 1-3

The tissue fates of the three germ layers of the trilaminar embryo. *(From Moore K, Persaud TVN: The developing human: clinically oriented embryology, ed 8, Philadelphia, 2008, WB Saunders.)*

sclerotomes produce only seven cervical vertebrae (**N161; G4.50; GY44; C356**)?

INTERVERTEBRAL DISCS

(N155, 162; G4.17; GY 32, 33; C351, 352)

Sclerotome cells lying diffusely between adjacent vertebral bodies form concentric layers of fibrocartilaginous connective tissue surrounding the notochord. These cells become the **annulus fibrosus** of the intervertebral disc. The gelatinous core of the disc, the **nucleus pulposus,** is composed, in part, of the remnant of the notocord. The reduction in disc height and loss of elasticity with age is associated with desiccation (loss of water) of the intervertebral disc and begins at approximately age 30. Weakening or tears of the annulus fibrosus may result in protrusion or frank extrusion of the nucleus pulposus. This event is called a disc herniation and occurs most frequently in the lumbar region of the spine at the posterolateral aspect of the disc. *What associated structures and what aspects of range of motion influence the location of disc herniations?*

TYPICAL VERTEBRA

The vertebral column normally consists of a total of 33 vertebrae: 7 cervical, 12 thoracic, 5 lumbar, 5 sacral, and 4 coccygeal (**N153; G4.3, 4.4; GY21, 22; C436**). Although each vertebral region has specialized features, all are derived from the primitive pattern of the thoracic vertebrae (**N147; G4.4; GY26, 27; C347**):

- A weight-bearing part—the vertebral body
- A part that protects the spinal cord—the neural arch, which consists of the pedicles and laminae
- Three levers for muscle attachment—the spinous process and right and left transverse processes
- Four points of articulation with adjacent vertebrae—two superior and two inferior articular processes, or zygapophyses

Although they may differ in size and shape from region to region, homologies can be drawn between the corresponding parts of regional vertebrae (**G4.5**): (Figure 1-4). Note especially the presence of a rudimentary rib element in regions that typically do not have ribs.

Body

The vertebral bodies contribute approximately 75% of the length of the presacral vertebral column; the remaining 25% added by the thickness of the intervertebral discs. Note that the vertebral bodies increase in thickness and width from cervical to lumbar regions, reflecting their weight-bearing function. The generalized cross-sectional outlines of the vertebral bodies differ regionally. In the cervical region, the vertebral bodies are elliptical (**N18; G4.9; GY22, 24**); in the thoracic region they are heart-shaped (**N154; G4.15; GY26; C347**); in the lumbar region they are kidney-bean-shaped (**N155; G4.16; GY29; C350**). The first cervical vertebra, the **atlas** (**N17; G4.12; GY24; C342**), has no body. In its place is the **dens,** a bony projection from the second cervical vertebra, the **axis.**

Vertebral Arch

The vertebral arches enclose the **vertebral foramina,** which in series form the **vertebral canal** (**N154; G4.4; GY22; C347**), housing the spinal cord and its coverings. The size of the canal varies regionally, being largest in the cervical region, narrowing in the thoracic region, and enlarging slightly again in the lumbar region. A broad generalization can also be made regarding the shape of the vertebral canal in each region of the vertebral column. In the cervical region the canal tends to be large and oval to accommodate the cervical enlargement; in the thoracic region, it is smaller and pentagonal; in the lumbar region, it is large and roughly triangular. Because the pedicles are narrower than the vertebral bodies, when viewed in

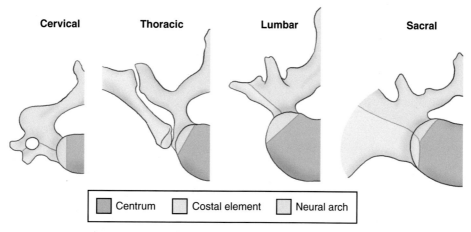

Cervical   Thoracic   Lumbar   Sacral

☐ Centrum   ☐ Costal element   ☐ Neural arch

FIGURE 1-4

Homologies expressed between vertebra and individual spinal levels. Note especially the costal element is present in all vertebral levels.

lateral perspective, notches lie superior and inferior to the pedicles. The inferior notch is the deeper of the two. In juxtaposed vertebrae, the superior and inferior vertebral notches form the **intervertebral foramen,** which permits the egress of the spinal nerve. The two halves of the **laminae** fuse in the midline, forming the roof of the vertebral canal. Note the rugosities (roughened surfaces) on the superior and inferior borders of the laminae, corresponding to the attachment of the

Clinical Note

Spina bifida occulta

Malformations involving the closure of the neural tube are collectively called **spina bifida.** They tend to be located at either the cervical or the caudal ends of the vertebral column. Why? (Failed closure of the cranial end of the neural tube results in anencephaly.)

   The mildest form of spina bifida is called spina bifida occulta. The neural arch has two primary centers of ossification. Failure of these areas to fuse completely results in an incomplete lamina, usually at L5 and or S1. This defect is present in up to 24% of the population. However, it is concealed beneath the skin, although its presence is often betrayed by a tuft of hair, pigmented nevus, or dimple. In most cases the meninges and spinal cord are normal, and the defect is asymptomatic. If more than one lumbar vertebrae are involved, the frequency of low back pain is greater (Figure 1-5).

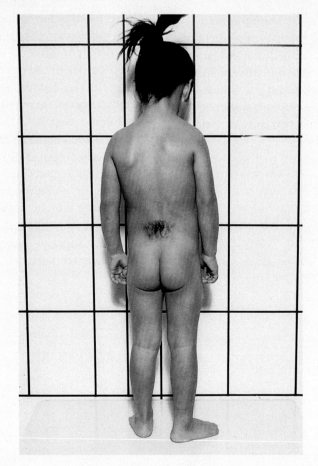

FIGURE 1-5
An infant with a hairy patch in the lumbosacral region, indicating the site of a spina bifida occulta. *(Courtesy of AE Chudley, MD, Section of Genetics and Metabolism, Department of Pediatrics and Child Health, Children's Hospital and University of Manitoba, Winnipeg, Manitoba, Canada. From Moore K, Persaud TVN:* Before we are born: essentials of embryology and birth defects, *ed 7, Philadelphia, 2008, WB Saunders.)*

ligamenta flava (N158; G4.18, 4.19; GY35; C351). This ligament is composed of **fibroelastic connective tissue** and is extremely important for limiting excessive flexion of the vertebral column.

Spinous Process

Because no powerful back muscles reach the atlas, it has no spinous process, merely a **posterior tubercle** (N17; G4.12; GY24; C342) for attachment of the **ligamentum nuchae.** Vertebrae C2 through C6 have short bifid (forked) spinous processes. These vertebrae are sometimes palpable but are usually obscured by the ligamentum nuchae (N21; G4.10; GY35), a fibrous triangular ligament spanning from the **external occipital protuberance,** the spinous process of C7, and the spinous processes of the remaining cervical vertebrae. Flex your neck and run your finger inferiorly along the ligamentum nuchae. The first bony protuberance encountered is the spinous process of the C7 vertebra, known as the **vertebral prominens** (N21; G4.11; GY23). C7 is a transitional vertebra, and its spinous process is not bifid. This area is a useful reference point for counting thoracic vertebrae. On a partner, locate the spinous process of T7 by counting down from the vertebral prominens. It should roughly correspond to the **scapular line,** a horizontal line drawn between the inferior angles of the scapulae. The thoracic spinous processes are much longer than the cervical or lumbar and are angled more inferiorly (N154, 155; G4.15; GY26, 28), which is especially the case with the middle one third of the thoracic region, T5 through T8. The spinous processes of the lumbar vertebrae are short, quadrangular, and nearly horizontal. The spinous process of L4 coincides with the **intercristal line,** a line between the highest points of the crest of the ilium.

Transverse Processes

Transverse processes are lever-like projections that extend from the sides of the vertebral arch. Anterior to the transverse process is the **costal element** (G4.5). In the thoracic region the costal element is extremely elongated and forms the rib. In cervical, lumbar, and sacral regions, the costal element is fused to the transverse process and does not usually extend significantly into the body wall. Occasionally a cervical or lumbar rib develops (N181; G1.14). **Lumbar ribs** are rarely symptomatic, but **cervical ribs** may cause clinical symptoms arising from the compression of the **subclavian artery,** the **brachial plexus,** or both.

Between the transverse and costal elements of the cervical transverse processes is a gap. This gap is called the **transverse foramen,** which conveys the **vertebral artery.** The thoracic transverse processes bear costal facets for articulation with the tubercle of the rib. The lumbar transverse processes consist largely of the costal element, with the **mammillary process** and **accessory process** representing the true transverse element. A large portion of the **ala** of the sacrum consists of the costal elements.

Articular Processes
(N154; G4.4; GY26)

Left and right articular facets are supported by the superior articular processes, or zygapophyses, and two facets are supported by the inferior zygapophyses. Note the change in the orientation of the articular facets as you proceed caudally along the spine. Their orientations grade from relatively horizontal to coronal to parasagittal. *How do these orientations differentially limit movements in the respective regions of the vertebral column?* Relate this observation to your explanation of the appearance of the hump in the case of scoliosis.

SACRUM
(N157; G4.23, 4.24; GY31; C353)

The sacrum is typically composed of five fused vertebrae. The fusion of the spinous processes produces the **median sacral crest.** The fused transverse processes form the **lateral sacral crest,** and the bumps formed by the articular processes form the **intermediate sacral crest.**

COCCYX
(N157; G4.23, 4.24; GY31; C353)

The coccyx, or tailbone, has no weight-bearing function and only a single coccygeal spinal nerve. It consists of four rudiments of vertebral bodies and no vertebral arches. Men frequently have an additional coccygeal element; women frequently have fewer. Fusion is usually delayed in women, as might be expected given the demands of parturition (childbirth) for an unobstructed pelvic outlet.

PRIMARY AND SECONDARY CURVATURES
(N153; G4.2; GY21; C346)

At birth the entire vertebral column has a **primary curve** that is concave on its ventral surface. This primary curvature persists into adulthood in the thoracic and sacral regions. An extreme condition of this thoracic curvature is known as a **kyphosis.** *Can you detect any differences in the anterior versus posterior height of the vertebral bodies in the thoracic region?* The sacral curvature in women is less marked than in men such that the sacrum impinges less on the pelvic outlet, or birth canal. The **secondary curves** develop as a response to upright posture and are found in the cervical and lumbar regions. The curves are convex on the ventral surface **(lordosis).** The cervical lordosis develops as the infant begins to hold the head up. The lumbar lordosis develops as the infant begins to stand and walk.

Examine radiographs of the normal spine and note the relationships of the vertebral bodies in various regions (N13, 156, 213; G4.7, 4.8, 4.16, 4.21; GY23, 27, 28, 29; C354, 355).

Exercises

1. In preparation for your first dissection, draw in and number the dermatomes on the figure of the back. Indicate the location of the vertebral prominence, the scapular line, and the intercristal line. To what dermatomes do these landmarks correspond?

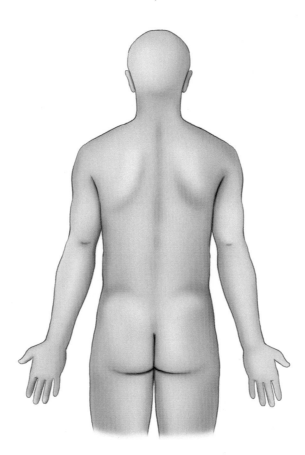

2. Measure and chart on the graph below the measured heights of the vertebral bodies. Explain the pattern you observe in the two lines.

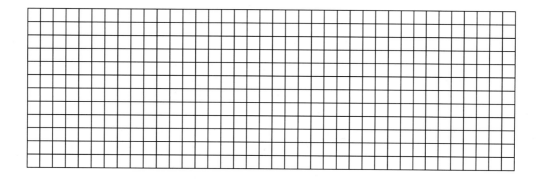

3. Extra ribs in the lumbar region generally are of little consequence. Cervical ribs, however, can be symptomatic. What visceral structures pass cranial to the first thoracic rib and inferior to the clavicle that might be impinged by a cervical rib? Color in the costal element of the cervical vertebra below.

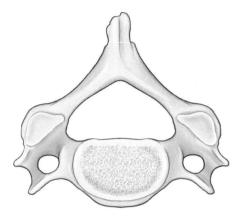

4. What generalizations can be made about the orientation of the articular surfaces of the zygapophyses? Why is L1 called the transitional vertebra?

5. Flexibility and strength of back muscles are helpful in the management of scoliosis. What muscles may be in imbalance and what type of exercises might prove effective in treating symptoms of back pain and fatigue?

Back

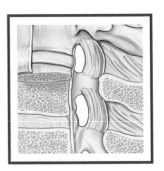

CASE STUDY

Spring Clean-Up

Jack is a 50 **y/o** college professor coming to the local clinic for an evaluation 3 days after he felt pain pulling weeds and doing yard work over the first warm weekend of spring. He indicates that it took him approximately 3 hours of steady work to get the yard in shape and he felt a bit "fatigued." He awoke the next morning with a substantial level of pain in the upper back area and had difficulty getting out of bed and performing general activities around the house. He self-medicated with over-the-counter **(OTC)** antiinflammatory and pain medications, which seemed to help little to alleviate the signs and symptoms. Today, Jack has pain and spasm in the shoulders and upper aspects of the back, and he suggests that the pain has actually increased and that his back and arm

muscles feel painful even to touch. His **PMH** and **systems review** is negative for significant disease. Jack is active and maintains a consistent exercise training regimen. He wants to run in an upcoming local marathon and is concerned that he will not be able to train appropriately with this pain. His active range of motion **(AROM)**, gross muscle strength, and dermatomes are intact in bilateral (B) upper extremities. Although Jack does complain of pain on all movements, he has little pain when the joints are moved passively by the examiner. The pain does not appear to be musculature.

Identification of the Anatomy

Identify structures in the various regions of the vertebral column. Focus on bony landmarks, muscle, and connective tissues, including posterior aspects of the scapula, such as the acromio-clavicular joint, spine, and inferior and medial angle.

Appreciate the following structures during dissection:

Superficial fascia

Major muscles of the posterior shoulder girdle and
    thorax

   Rhomboideus major and minor

   Levator scapulae

   Trapezius

   Serratus anterior

   Latissimus dorsi

   Thoracodorsal aponeurosis

   Rhomboideus Trapezius

Questions

1. Can you postulate why the signs and symptoms are getting worse over a 3-day period?
2. Why does this patient feel less pain when the examiner moves his arms passively as opposed to when Jack moves his arm himself? What types of conditions refer pain to the low back?
3. What is the relationship of the gait abnormality to the pathologic condition of the spine?

Discussion

Jack has the classic signs and symptoms of overuse injury. The concepts of specificity of muscle movement and training are both applicable. Muscles generally need a progressive resistance for conditioning, and Jack has a condition known as delayed onset of muscle soreness **(DOMS)**. This condition results from overusing and stressing muscle tissue, which causes damage to the cellular matrix of the muscle and leads to an increase in pressure secondary to cell or connective-tissue damage, altering fluid dynamics within the muscle and surrounding tissues and thus causing pain. The signs and symptoms generally subside with time and the introduction of progressive training of the muscle. Furthermore, eccentrical muscle loading (tension of the muscle during lengthening) seems to cause the condition more frequently than concentric (muscle shortening during tension). Because the muscle is swollen (edema), even tactile pressure may increase local pain.

Preparation

Have an articulated skeleton present to assist with your determination of joint shape and movements, muscle attachments, and assessments of muscle action. A sharp scalpel blade is essential for effective dissection technique. Do not scrimp! The extensive incisions and thickness of the skin on the back will dull your blade rapidly. Receive instructions for changing blades safely, and refresh your blade as needed.

Anatomic Overview

The study of joints is termed **arthrology.** A functional definition of a joint is a gap between two bones developed for the purpose of permitting motion between them. Joints are also involved in the union of two osseous elements of a bone in such a way as to provide for continued growth. Two major schemes exist for classifying the variety of joints present in the human body.

STRUCTURAL CLASSIFICATION

The first classification scheme is based on the *structure* and nature of the tissues uniting the two skeletal elements. Three classes are represented: fibrous, cartilaginous, and synovial (Figure 2-1).

   Fibrous joints are united by fibrous connective tissue, and the potential for movement is usually quite restricted. These joints include three types: first, the interlocking **suture** joints of the cranium; second, the peglike **gomphoses** of the tooth and alveolus; third, the lashing-like **syndesmoses** of, for example, the distal tibiofibular joint.

   Cartilaginous joints are united either by hyaline cartilage or by fibrocartilage. Those joined by hyaline cartilage are called **synchondroses.** These structures are temporary joints representing the growth plate or **epiphyseal plate** uniting two centers of ossification. On maturation the joint is obliterated and becomes a **synostosis. Symphyses** are joints joined by an intervening fibrocartilaginous pad or plate, as is found in the intervertebral disc or the symphysis pubis.

   Synovial joints are by far the most common throughout the body. The ends of the articulated bones are covered with **hyaline cartilage** and enclosed by a **fibrous joint capsule** reinforced with ligaments. The capsule is lined by a **synovial membrane** that produces the **synovial fluid.** Frequently, fibrocartilaginous discs or menisci are found within the joint capsule (Figure 2-2).

FUNCTIONAL CLASSIFICATION

The second classification scheme is based on the *function* or potential movements of the joints. The amount of movement is determined by the joint shape and can also be defined by the axes of rotation.

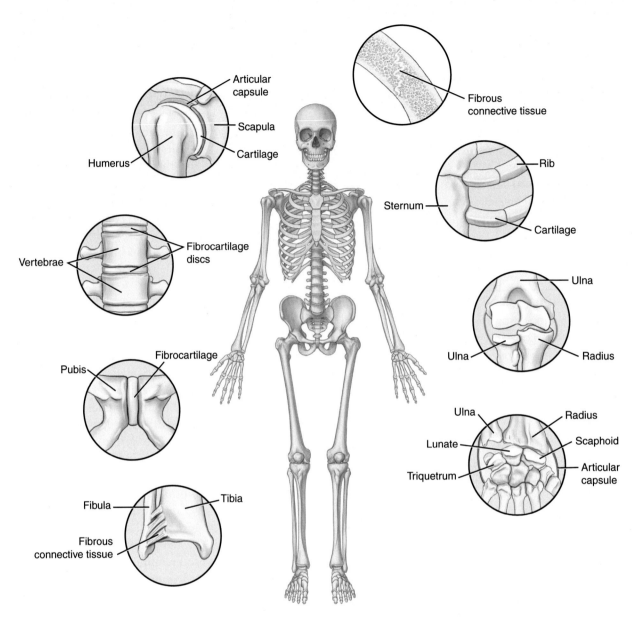

FIGURE 2-1
Examples of joints found throughout the skeleton. *(Modified from Drake R et al:* Gray's anatomy for students, *Philadelphia, 2005, Churchill Livingstone.)*

Synarthroses

Also known as *skull-type* joints, synarthroses are represented by the sutures in the skull. Because of the limited movement, the adjacent bones essentially act as one (Gr. *syn* = same).

Amphiarthroses

Amphiarthroses, also known as *vertebral-type* joints, lie in the median plane and include intervertebral discs and the symphysis pubis. These joints permit a moderate range of movement (Gr. *amphi* = on both sides; about).

Diarthroses

Diarthroses are the most common joints in the body and are known as *limb-type* joints, although examples are also found in the axial skeleton. These joints are highly moveable (Gr. *di* = two). Diarthroses are further subdivided based on the shape of the articular surfaces. Locate and write in an example of each of the following shapes:

Planar _____

Hinge _____

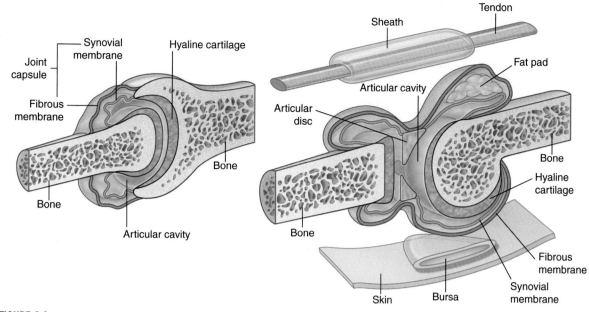

FIGURE 2-2
Components of synovial joints, synovial sheaths, and bursa. (*From Drake R et al:* Gray's anatomy for students, *Philadelphia, 2005, Churchill Livingstone.*)

Pivot _____

Saddle _____

Condyloid _____

Ball and socket _____

The shape of the joint in turn constrains the **axis** (or **axes**) **of rotation.** The axes of rotation are the pivot points about which movements occur. Joints can be nonaxial, uniaxial, biaxial, and multiaxial.

Typical vertebrae are united to each other by three types of joints: symphysis (intervertebral discs), syndesmoses (longitudinal ligaments, ligamentum flavum, interspinous and supraspinous ligaments), and synovial (zygapophyses) (Figure 2-3).

LIGAMENTS
(N158, 159; G4.18, 4.19; GY35; C350, 351)
Several ligaments span the intervertebral spaces, thus linking adjacent vertebrae.

Anterior and posterior longitudinal ligaments
Ligamentum flavum
Interspinous and supraspinous ligaments
Intertransverse ligaments

MOVEMENTS
Movements of the vertebral column are defined in relation to anatomic position.

Flexion—reduction of joint angle from 180° (i.e., forward bending)
Extension—increase in joint angle to 180° in the sagittal plane
Hyperextension—extension beyond 180°
Lateral flexion—bending in the frontal plane
Rotation—twisting about the long axis

Which of the foregoing ligaments limit flexion? Which limit extension?

ASSESSING MUSCLE ACTION
What follows is a series of steps that will permit you to determine the action of any muscle without resorting to rote memorization. These steps are as follows:

1. Identify the muscle attachments.
2. Identify the joint or joints crossed by the muscle.
3. Determine the axis or axes of rotation of the joint in question.
4. Assess muscle action as determined by the line of pull of the muscle relative to the axis or axes of rotation.

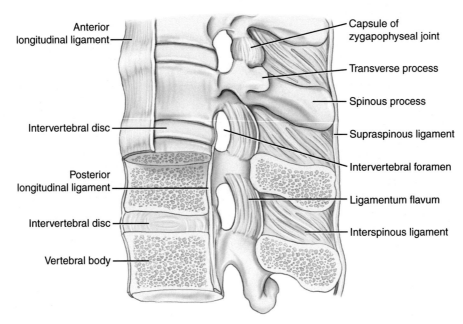

FIGURE 2-3
Intervertebral joints. Note that two adjacent vertebrae and the intervening intervertebral disc constitute the *functional unit* of the spine.

Take as an example the transversospinalis muscle group. The assessment of muscle action would proceed as follows:

- Attachments: from the transverse processes to the spinous processes above
- Joints crossed: intervertebral

- Axes of rotation: represented by the intersection of any two anatomic planes
  a. Transverse axis (intersection of the frontal and horizontal planes), permitting flexion-extension in the sagittal plane (Figure 2-4, *A*)
  b. Anterior-posterior (AP) axis (intersection of the sagittal and horizontal planes),

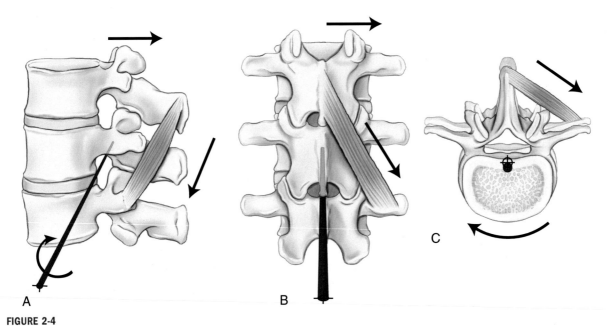

FIGURE 2-4
A, Extension occurs about the transverse axis of rotation. **B,** Lateral bending occurs about an anterior-posterior axis of rotation. **C,** Rotation occurs about a vertical axis of rotation.

permitting abduction-adduction in the coronal plane (Figure 2-4, *B*)

   c. Vertical axis (intersection of the frontal and sagittal planes), permitting rotation in the horizontal plane (Figure 2-4, *C*).

- Actions:
  - Transverse axis: line of pull passes behind the transverse axis, producing extension
  - AP axis: line of pull is lateral to the AP axis, producing lateral bending
  - Vertical axis: line of pull is posterior to the longitudinal axis such that the transversospinalis exert rotation of the trunk
- Summary: the transversospinalis extend, laterally bend, and rotate the truck.

EMBRYOGENESIS OF DERMOMYOTOMES

You may recall that each somite differentiated into a sclerotome, which gave rise to the vertebrae, and a dermomyotome, which contained the precursor cells for the dermis and skeletal muscles. Each dermomyotome then divides into a small **epaxial dermomyotome** (or epimere) and a larger **hypaxial dermomyotome** (or hypomere) (Figure 2-5). Muscles derived from the epaxial dermomyotomes constitute the intrinsic muscles of the back and are innervated by **dorsal rami** of spinal nerves.

The remaining back muscles are derived from hypaxial dermomyotomes or **cranial somite** cells that have migrated into the back. These muscles are not innervated by dorsal rami of spinal nerves but rather by **ventral rami** of spinal nerves or branches of cranial nerves, respectively.

Dissection

Place the cadaver prone (face down), and place a block under the chest so that the neck can be flexed forward.

Palpate the following bony landmarks:
   External occipital protuberance (inion)
   Mastoid process
   Vertebral prominens
   Vertebral border of the scapula and scapular spine
   Acromion process
   Iliac crest
   Posterior-superior iliac spine

A thorough knowledge of the topographic relationships of underlying soft tissues to superficial bony landmarks is important. The skin of the cadaver is not as pliable as living tissue; hence palpation instructions should also be carried out on yourself or a partner.

Make an incision along the midline from just above the inion to coccyx.

Make transverse incisions from the vertebral prominens to the acromion process, from T7 along the scapular line, and finally from the coccyx along the iliac crest taking care to gauge the depth of the incision. (Additional transverse incisions may be added as needed for convenience of skin reflection.)

As incisions are made, the scalpel blade will encounter several layers of tissue. The epidermis

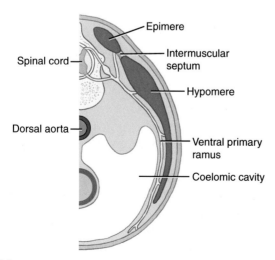
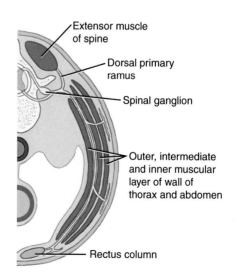

FIGURE 2-5
The fate of the hypomere in forming the muscles of the body wall.

and dermis are of variable thickness (1 to 2 mm), depending on the region and age of the individual. The skin on the back is generally rather thick. Beneath the skin is the hypodermis, a layer of **loose irregular connective tissue** (or **areolar tissue**), known by gross anatomists as the **superficial fascia** (Figure 2-6). The superficial fascia is a repository of fat cells distributed throughout the body, except for the glans of the penis and clitoris. Fibrocysts form a network with their long, thin processes. A latticework of interconnected collagen fibers lends tensile strength to the tissue, whereas branching elastic fibers produce elasticity, allowing distorted tissue to return to its original shape. Cutaneous nerves and vessels often run for considerable distance within the superficial fascia and will be encountered here. The superficial fascia is loosely anchored to the underlying tissue by collagen fibers. Beneath the superficial fascia is a layer of **dense irregular connective tissue** that invests the muscle. Histologists refer to this tissue as the **epimysium;** gross anatomists call it the **deep fascia.** Here the density of collagen fibers is arrayed in feltlike fashion, that is, no dominant orientation to the fibers. Thus it has tensile strength in all directions (Figure 2-7).

TIP To reflect the skin flaps, begin at a corner, that is, the intersection of a midline and transverse incision. Initially, avoid the skin and fascia over the nape of the neck, which can be quite thick and fibrous. Reflect the corner far enough that you can make a stab incision, similar to a buttonhole through the skin, large enough to accommodate your index finger (see Figure 1-3). Next, apply firm tension on the flap and draw the scalpel, with the blade held horizontally, across the stretched collagen fibers anchoring the superficial fascia to the deep fascia. Note the inverse relationship between the force applied and the skin flap and the force applied to the scalpel to detach the skin.

Watch for the emergence of neurovascular bundles (**N177; G4.3; GY17; C338**) through the deep fascia within a few centimeters of the midline as the skin and superficial fascia are being reflected.
Save short segments of several of these for review. The neural components of these bundles are the

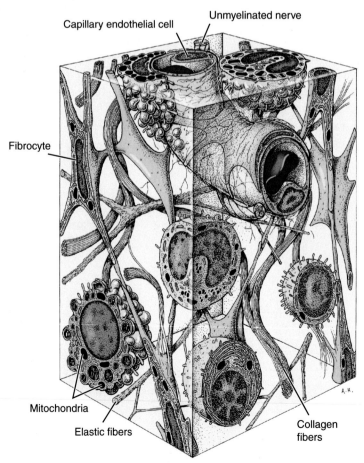

Capillary endothelial cell

Unmyelinated nerve

Fibrocyte

Mitochondria

Elastic fibers

Collagen fibers

FIGURE 2-6
Structural histology of superficial fascia. (*Modified from Krstic RV: General histology of the mammal, Berlin, 1984, Springer-Verlag.*)

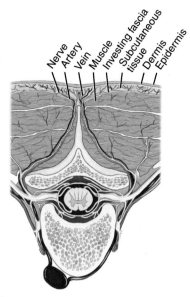

FIGURE 2-7
Transverse section showing the course of a neurovascular bundle traversing the deep and superficial fascias in the epaxial region of the back.

cutaneous nerve branches of the dorsal rami of spinal nerves (N192; G1.18; GY 72; C327).

Superficial Muscle Layer

(N174; G4.28; GY37, 38; C328)

The first muscles encountered are **extrinsic back muscles;** that is, they attach to the pectoral girdle or limb skeleton. These muscles are the trapezius and the latissimus dorsi. Notice that they cover almost the entire back.

Clean the surface of the muscles, and determine the orientation of their fibers and their attachments.

Trapezius (spinal accessory n., CN XI: occipital somites; hypaxial myotomes: C3, 4).
A composite muscle derived from occipital somites and hypaxial dermomyotomes C3, 4.

> **TIP** Near the cranial attachment of the trapezius, locate the dorsal ramus of C2, the greater occipital nerve, as it emerges through the deep fascia near the occipital artery.

Latissimus dorsi (thoracodorsal n. C6, 7, 8; also known as the middle subscapular or nerve to latissimus dorsi).
The latissimus dorsi is a hypaxial muscle of the upper limb.

Cut the trapezius along the spinous processes and superior nuchal line, reflecting it toward its attachment along the clavicle.

Cut the thoracolumbar fascia, and reflect the muscle laterally.
Identify each of the muscle groups below, and assess their functions as previously outlined.

Intermediate muscle layer

(N177; G4.32; GY39; C332)
Rhomboideus major and minor (**dorsal scapular n., C5**)
Levator scapulae (C3, 4, [5])
Serratus posterior inferior et. superior

Deep muscle layer c

(N176, G4.33, 4.35; GY40, 41; C333) This layer consists of the intrinsic back muscles, innervated by local branches of spinal nerves, and function in maintenance of posture and movement.
Splenius cervicus et. capitus (C2-5; C9-12)
Erector spinae (dorsal rami of local spinal nerves)
Spinalis
Longissimus
Iliocostalis
Transversospinalis (dorsal rami of local spinal nerves)
Rotatores (span one to two segments); most developed in the thoracic region
Semispinalis cervicus et. capitus (span four to six segments)
Multifidus (span three to five segments); most pronounced in the lumbar region where they arise from the mammillary bodies

Clinical Note

Spare your back—proper lifting

Electromyographic studies of the intrinsic back muscles reveal that they are relatively inactive when standing at ease. *What anatomic features of the vertebral column hold the torso upright without muscular effort?* Through eccentric contraction, the erector spinae control the rate of forward bending. However, when a certain degree of full flexion is attained, the erector spinae relax, and the strain is taken up by the ligaments of the vertebral column and the various facet joints. When lifting a load from this position, the erector spinae remain inactive at first, the initial stage of extension being carried out by the hamstrings and gluteus maximus, retractors of the hip. This action places tremendous strain on the ligaments of the back, potentially causing injurious sprains and inflammation of these connective tissues. Muscles of the back may go into spasm as a protective mechanism if the back is thus injured. *What is the anatomic basis of proper lifting?*

Exercises

1. Describe the shape and indicate the axis or axes of rotation for each of the figured joints.

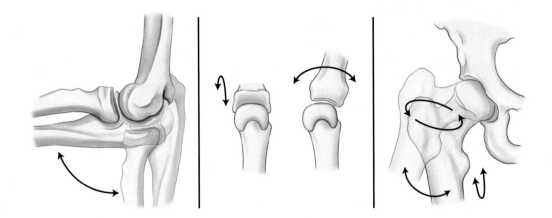

2. What are the three types of joints found in the back? Name them according to a structural and functional classification scheme.

Joint	Structural	Functional

3. Draw in and label the ligaments of the syndesmoses of the back. What movements do they restrict?

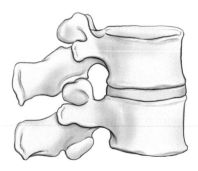

4. On the figure of the back skeleton, draw in simple lines between the points of attachment of the erector spinae muscle group on the left and the transversospinalis group on the right.

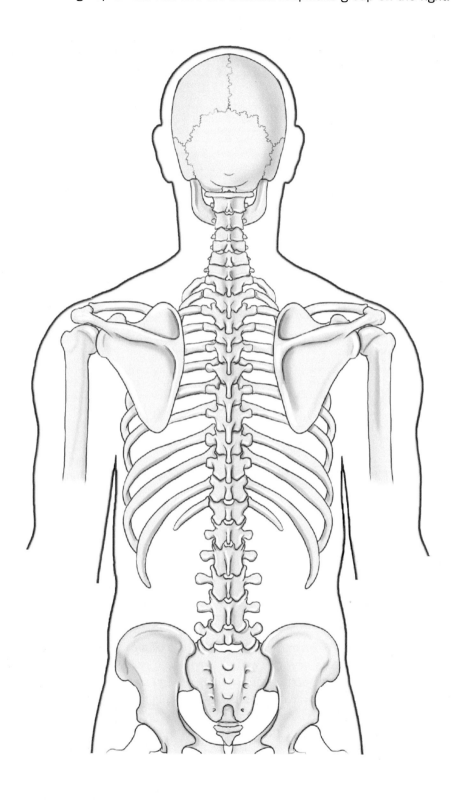

LAB EXPLORATION **3**

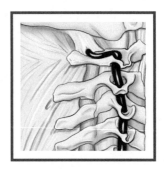

Suboccipital Triangle

LAB OBJECTIVES

This lab considers a small field of dissection that encompasses the posterior muscles that attach the vertebral column to the head. The mass of the head places stress on these structures. When you have completed this lab exploration, you should be able to:

- Define the boundaries and describe the contents of the suboccipital triangle.
- Trace the path of the vertebral artery.
- Name and describe the distribution of the first three dorsal rami of cervical spinal nerves.
- Assess the actions of the epaxial muscles of the neck.

CASE STUDY

Whiplash

Melanie, who is a 62 **y/o** retired woman, visits your outpatient **(O.P.)** rehabilitation clinic as a referral from a local medical doctor **(LMD)** with a request to evaluate and treat the patient for neck pain and headaches (HA). Melanie is a very active woman and indicates her main **c/o** pain is related to her neck during her exercise activity, which includes cross-country skiing, swimming, and a vigorous walking program. She indicates that she exercises three times a week (3 x wk.), and the pain forms ultimately into a suboccipital origin headache and pain in rotation of the head after exercise. The discomfort lasts for several hours and is relieved by taking nonsteroidal antiinflammatory drugs **(NSAID)**. The examination reveals marked decrease of **A/PROM** in rotation and initial flexion and extension of the head. Side-bending of the cervical spine is **WNL**. Frank **crepitus** is noted in all directions of motion in the cervical region. Melanie complains of exquisite pain on rotation over pressure to the **R** and **L**. Her vertebral artery test

was negative. The **PMH** indicates that she suffered a whiplash injury in a **MVA** after which she was immobilized with a cervical brace for 6 weeks as a result of the pain she suffered during the hyperextension of the neck.

Identification of the Anatomy

The upper and lower regions of the cervical vertebral column are extremely important in relation to head motions in all functional planes. The anatomy of the atlantooccipital joint complex, occiput, C1-C2, and the levels of C2 through C7 are crucial to the understanding of movement in the cervical spine, given that this area of the column has the greatest motion in rotation and lateral side-bending. The structure of the vertebra and the soft tissues give this area great mobility with little stability.

Appreciate the following structures during dissection:

Muscle and ligament structures
    Overlying: trapezius, splenius, semispinalis capitus
    Deep: superior oblique, inferior oblique, rectus
       major and rectus minor

Tectorial membrane, alar ligament, cruciform ligament complex, apical dental ligament (Observe the ligaments in your atlas, N17, 18; G4.14. They will be considered in the cadaver in a later exploration.)

Nerve

Greater occipital nerve and associated branches

Vertebrae and occiput

C1: (atlas) arch, posterior tubercle and facet joints

C2: (axis) dens, transverse foramen

C3-C7: facet joints, transverse foramen, intervertebral discs

Questions

1. Given the current signs and symptoms of this patient, what might be the cause of the pain and headaches?
2. Why would the pain increase after exercise?
3. What function is served by the atypical arrangement of the atlantoaxial joint?

Discussion

The structure of the cervical spine and surrounding tissues is designed to allow total **ROM** of the head of approximately 160 degrees of rotation, 90 degrees of side-bending, and 90 in flexion and extension. Approximately 90 degrees of range in rotation occurs at the C1-C2 segment, with the rest being taken up by the lower segments C3 through C7. The noticeable **crepitus** (abnormal joint grinding sound secondary to worn surfaces) may be the result of gradual use and wear and tear of the joint surfaces (degenerative joint disease) over the last 30 years. Her joint pain and decrease in **ROM** are secondary to this gradual loss of function with associated joint capsule stiffness. The greater occipital nerve emerges just inferior to the suboccipital triangle, communicates with the suboccipital nerve, and its branches course into various supporting musculature of the head. This arrangement, coupled with the increased blood circulation and active **ROM** of the head and upper back during exercise, may be the cause of the headaches after exercise. The relief of symptoms through **NSAID** use is consistent with decreasing the inflammation in associated joints and muscles.

Preparation

On the skeleton, identify the **superior nuchal lines, foramen magnum, posterior tubercle,** and the **foramen transversarum** of the atlas and the **spinous process** and **transverse foramen** of the

axis. The muscles and the ligaments of this region are associated with the **atlantooccipital** and **atlantoaxial** joints. These joints are significant for the flexion-extension and rotation of the head on the vertebral column. The extreme range of rotation of the head about the neck occurs largely at the atlantoaxial joint (Figure 3-1). Review the specialized anatomy of the first two cervical vertebrae (N17, 22; G4.9, 4.12; GY24; C342, 344). Their anatomy and associated ligaments will be examined in greater detail in a subsequent lab.

Anatomic Overview

The craniovertebral muscles act on the head by extending it on C1 at the atlantooccipital joints or rotating it between C1 and C2 at the atlantoaxial joints. Larger muscles have similar actions (e.g., the trapezius, splenius capitus, sternocleidomastoid). Smaller muscles of pairs with similar action may serve as proprioceptive organs, providing a sense of position for the cranium relative to the vertebral column.

The appearance of muscle is a grainy texture. This grain is the result of muscle fibers organized into fascicles. To appreciate better the structural basis of the grain of muscle, we will briefly consider the histogenesis and architecture of skeletal muscle. Embryonic cells of the myotome differentiate into myoblasts. These myoblasts align themselves end to end and fuse, losing the intervening cell membranes. This process produces a multinucleated syncytium, or shared cytoplasm. The myofiber begins to produce and organize the intracellular contractile proteins. Each muscle fiber is surrounded by a fine, loose connective tissue called the **endomysium** (Figure 3-2). Several fibers are encompassed by a slightly more substantial loose connective tissue, called the **perimysium.** Finally, the collection of fascicles constitutes the muscle belly, which is encompassed by the **epimysium,** or deep fascia, a layer of dense irregular connective tissue.

TIP One way to think of the relationship between the muscle fibers of a muscle belly and its connective tissue investments is a Chinese finger trap. The collagen fibers are the woven grass finger trap, and the muscle fibers are the fingers. As tension is applied to the fingers, as when muscle fibers contract, the trap tightens and produces more friction at their contact.

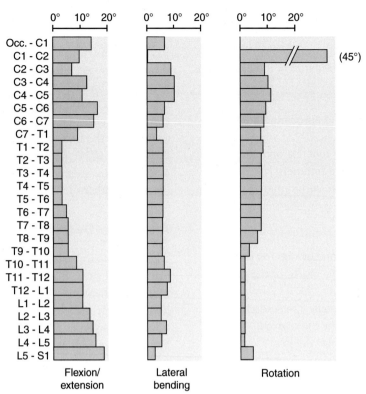

FIGURE 3-1
Typical ranges of motion at intervertebral and craniovertebral joints.

Dissection

Identify and **clean** the **splenius capitus** and **splenius cervicus, Detach** them from the spinous processes and **reflect** them laterally (**N175, 176; G4.33, 4.35; GY38, 39; C332**).

Identify the **semispinalis capitus** and **longissimus capitus.**

Detach the semispinalis capitus and longissimus capitus from the occipital bone, and **reflect** them inferiorly, taking care to preserve the **greater occipital nerve** (the medial branch of the dorsal ramus of C2 [**N178; G4.38; GY43; C341**]).

Follow the nerve to the inferior boundary of the suboccipital triangle (**N178; G4.39; GY43; C341**). The triangle is formed by the **inferior oblique, superior oblique,** and the **rectus capitus posterior major** (and **rectus capitus posterior minor**) muscles. Within the triangle, look for branches of the **suboccipital nerve** (dorsal ramus of C1).

Identify the **vertebral artery** (**N21; G4.39; GY43; C340**), and **palpate** the **posterior arch of the atlas.** Attempt to visualize the **atlantooccipital membrane.**

TIP The dissection field is frequently obscured by branches of the occipital and deep cervical veins. These branches must be removed to visualize the contents of the suboccipital triangle and adjacent structures. Also, note that the rectus capitus posterior major and minor are parallel but not coplanar. This arrangement is the result of the disparity in degree of posterior projection by the posterior tubercle of the posterior arch of the atlas and the spinous process of C2.

Review the courses of the dorsal rami of the first three cervical spinal nerves:

C1—suboccipital nerve. Innervates the suboccipital muscles and part of the semispinalis capitus. It often has no dorsal root because the sensory field is supplied by the greater occipital nerve.

C2—greater occipital nerve. Provides motor innervation to part of the semispinalis capitus and sensory innervation to the posterior scalp.

Notice the absence of C1 dermatome.

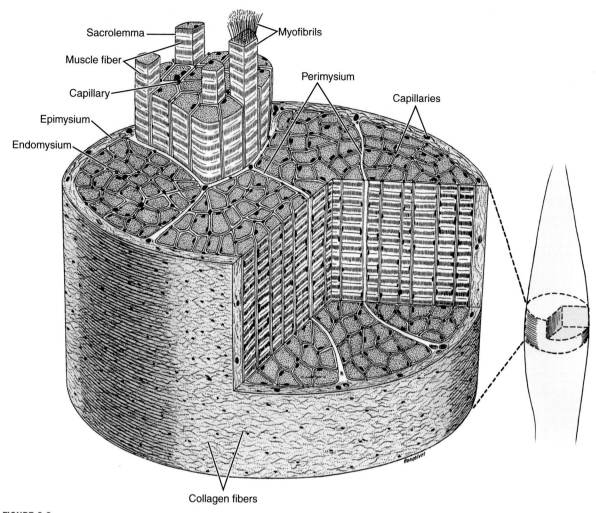

Sacrolemma

Myofibrils

Muscle fiber

Capillary

Perimysium

Epimysium

Capillaries

Endomysium

Collagen fibers

FIGURE 3-2

Cross-section of muscle belly illustrating its histological architecture. *(Modified from Junqueira LC, Carneiro J, Contopoulos AN: Basic histology, ed 2, Los Altos, California, 1977, Lang Medical Publications.)*

C3—third occipital nerve. Motor innervation to part of semispinalis capitus and sensory to the back of the neck up to the inion. (Note: This nerve should not be confused with the **lesser occipital nerve,** which is a branch of the cervical plexus formed by the *ventral* rami of C3 through C5.)

Assess the actions of the muscles of the suboccipital triangle employing the steps described in Lab Exploration 2.

Clinical Note

Vertebral artery insufficiency

Among the contents of the **suboccipital triangle** is the **vertebral artery.** It follows a serpentine route as it emerges from the foramen transversarum of the atlas (C1). It travels first posteriorly then medially on the superior surface of the **posterior arch** of the atlas, which is grooved by the artery. Here, the artery can be seen in the suboccipital triangle. It then passes beneath the **posterior atlantooccipital membrane (N17; C340)** (Figure 3-3). The free border of this membrane above the vertebral artery is called the **oblique ligament of the atlas** and becomes frequently ossified. The artery then turns upward, passing through the foramen magnum to enter the cranial cavity **(N130; C490)**.

   The tortuous path of the vertebral artery becomes clinically significant with hardening or narrowing of the artery, as in **arteriosclerosis**. Under these conditions, prolonged turning of the head, as when backing up the car, or resting the neck on the edge of a beauty salon sink, may cause dizziness or depression of brainstem functions as a result of vertebral artery insufficiency. Therapists may employ the *vertebral artery test* to suggest a perfusion insufficiency to the brain.

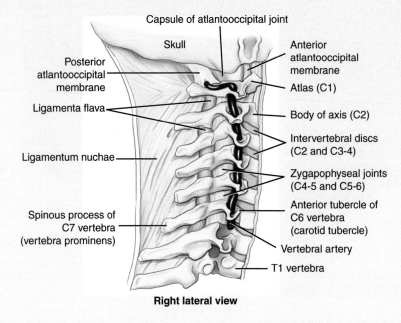

Right lateral view

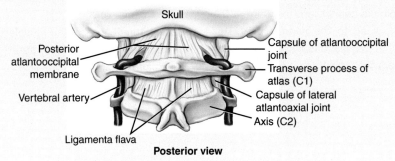

Posterior view

FIGURE 3-3

Ligaments and bony anatomy of the cervical spine (C1-C7), occipital triangle, and the course of the right and left vertebral arteries.

Exercises

1. On the figure below, indicate and label the dermatomes and the cutaneous nerve fields supplying the scalp and neck.

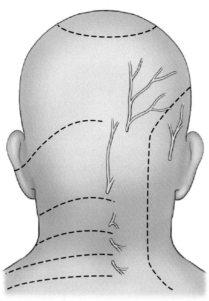

2. On the figure below indicate and label the boundaries of the suboccipital triangle and draw in the structures found within.

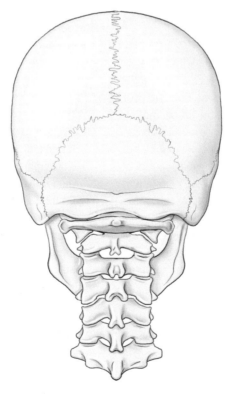

LAB EXPLORATION **4**

Spinal Cord

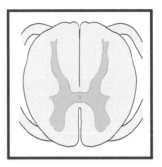

LAB OBJECTIVES

During this exploration, the spinal cord will be exposed within the vertebral canal by **laminectomy,** or removal of the vertebral laminae. On completion, you should be able to do the following:
- Identify the ligaments that restrict flexion of the vertebral column.
- Identify the coverings of the spinal cord and associated spaces.
- Identify the parts of the spinal cord and branches of the typical spinal nerve.

CASE STUDY

Leg Pain

Mr. Turner is a 54 **y/o** railroad engineer with a **BMI** of 35 who was seen 4 days ago by a physician in the **ER** for **LBP.** The patient stated that he was bending over to pick up a heavy toolbox when the lifting motion caused a sharp pain in his back, bringing him to his knees. He was able to complete his work shift but was unable to get up the next morning because of back pain and left lower extremity **(LLE)** pain and numbness. The patient had a **PMH** of **HTN,** past intermittent back pain, and 20 years of smoking one pack of cigarettes per day. On physical examination the physician noted a left positive **SLR** test, a decrease in the left **DTR** at L4, and a positive **CSR** on the same side; **B/B** symptoms were negative.

Identification of the Anatomy

The intervertebral discs, ribs, and overall structure play a major role in the stability and mobility of the column and in the functional protection of the spinal cord. The dissection of the vertebral column is difficult at best because of the complexity of overlying muscle and

connective tissue, especially via the posterior approach. The cervical, thoracic, lumbar, and sacral regions of the column are identified with their respective vertebral body number, size, and alterations in structure.

Appreciate the following structures during dissection:

Overlying musculature and tissue
   Superficial, intermediate, and deep muscular groupings
   Aponeuroses
Ligaments
   Longitudinal ligaments (anterior-posterior)
   Ligamentum nuchae
   Supraspinous ligaments
   Interspinous ligaments
Vertebrae (difference between regional characteristics)
   Spinous processes
   Transverse processes
   Vertebral canal
   Facet joints (zygapophysial)
   Pedicles
   Intervertebral foramen

Intervertebral discs
  Nucleus pulposus (NP)
  Annulus fibrosus (AF)
Spinal Cord
  Meninges
  Dorsal and ventral roots
  Dorsal root ganglion
Sympathetic chain ganglion

Questions

1. Given the patient's signs and symptoms during the examination, what is the cause of the problem?
2. Why are the symptoms occurring on the left side only?
3. Why does the **SLR** test evoke pain?

Discussion

The spine is extremely sensitive to loading in directions of flexion, extension, lateral side-bending, and rotation. This patient placed himself into position of disadvantage when he bent over to lift. The spine was in flexion and possible rotation, causing an abnormal force in the lumbar region, causing the L4-L5 disc to herniate and impinge on the left spinal nerve root where it emerged from the intervertebral foramen; hence the **radicular** sign is on the left side. The pain is only on the left side because the majority of disc herniation/protrusions occur posteriolaterally to the side of the posterior longitudinal, which is fused to and reinforces the central posterior portion of the annulus fibrosis of the intervertebral disc. The patient has a positive **SLR** test because the nerve root is stretched across the herniation when the leg is raised in the supine position. Even though these injuries do heal in time with bed rest and conservative treatment, some will ultimately need surgical intervention for symptom relief.

Preparation

Refer to the articulated vertebral column, and review the anatomy of the **vertebral arches** in the lower thoracic and lumbar spine (N148-151; G4.3; GY28, 29; C346, 347, 350). Note the disposition of the **laminae,** which form the roof of the vertebral canal. Locate the **intervertebral foramina** situated between adjacent **pedicles.** *What structure passes through the intervertebral foramen?*

Examine an isolated prossected spinal cord if one is available (N160; G4.41; GY45; C356, 357)

(Figure 4-1). Identify grey and white matter in cross-section (N169; G4.47; GY45). Note the **cervical** and **lumbosacral enlargements.** *Can you identify the dorsal and ventral roots and rootlets of the spinal nerves and identify the dorsal root ganglion and sympathetic chain ganglion* (N169, 170; G4.46; GY47; C359, 360)?

Anatomic Overview

In addition to structural support, the vertebral column provides protection for the spinal cord within the vertebral canal. The vertebral canal is formed by the series of successive **vertebral foramina** of the individual vertebrae. The spinal cord lies suspended within a fluid-filled sleeve of **dense fibrous connective tissue,** the **dura mater** (Figure 4-2).

The dura mater is continuous, with the **epineurium** surrounding the dorsal and ventral roots and the branches of the spinal nerve (Figure 4-3). The epineurium consists of strong, slightly undulating, longitudinally directed collagen fibers, which bind the **nerve fascicles** together, forming a nerve. The undulations of the collagen fibers lend some elasticity to the nerve. The individual fascicles are surrounded by the **perineurium,** which is continuous with the **arachnoid mater** of the central nervous system. The perineurium consists of several alternating laminae of flattened overlapping epithelial cells bound together by tight junctions. These laminae alternate with layers of longitudinally oriented collagen microfibrils. The multilaminar perineurium forms a selective diffusion barrier between the nerve fibers and the surrounding epineurial connective tissue. Within the fascicle are myelinated and unmyelinated nerve fibers, capillaries, and fibrocytes.

Dissection

Place the cadaver in prone position, and place a block under the pelvis to reduce the lumbar curve.

Review the arrangement of the **erector spinae** (N175; G4.33; GY40; C333). Then, if not already done, reflect them laterally to expose the **transversospinalis** muscles (N176; G4.35-37; GY41; C335). The transversospinalis muscles occupy the gutter formed by the spinous and transverse processes of the vertebrae (N179; G4.34; GY42; C327).

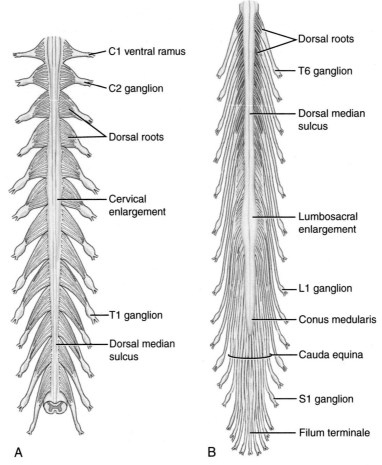

FIGURE 4-1
A, Cranial *(left)* and **B,** caudal *(right)* halves of the spinal cord.

Cut away piecemeal the transversospinalis between T6 and L5. As you do so, note the attachments, and identify fascicles of the individual groups.

Identify the **supraspinous ligament** and the **interspinous ligament,** which serve to restrict flexion of the vertebral column (**N158; G4.19; GY35; C351**). These ligaments are continuous with the ligamentum nuchae previously examined in the cervical region.

Use a scalpel to cut the interspinous ligaments.

LAMINECTOMY

Using bone snips, remove the spinous processes of the cleaned vertebrae to permit easier access with the bone saw.

Wearing protective goggles, use an oscillating bone saw to make an angled cut through the exposed laminae just medial to the zygapophyses (Figure 4-4). Take care to avoid cutting too deeply.

TIP The blade of the bone saw must be angled medially just enough to stay within the vertebral canal, otherwise the lamina will not be freed from the pedicles. If needed, the opening can be widened by removing additional bone. Hold the saw in one hand and brace it against the other to control the depth of penetration better. You can feel when the blade has passed through the bone. Note that the rounded saw blade requires that a side-to-side motion be made to complete the cut and free the laminae.

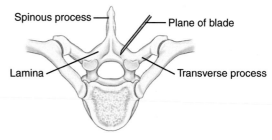

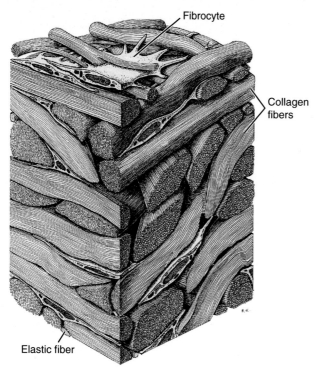

FIGURE 4-2
Dense irregular connective tissue. *(Modified from Krstic RV: General histology of the mammal, Berlin, 1984, Springer-Verlag.)*

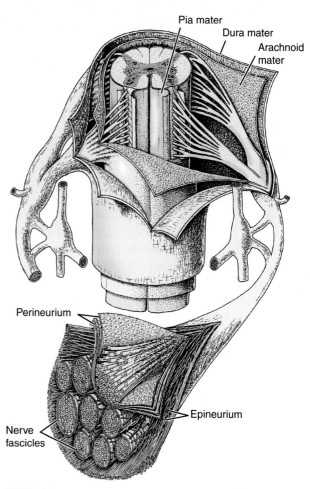

FIGURE 4-3
The coverings of the spinal cord and spinal nerves. *(Modified from Krstic RV: General histology of the mammal, Berlin, 1984, Springer-Verlag.)*

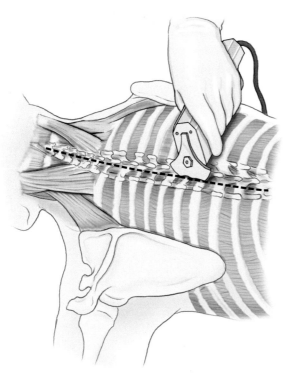

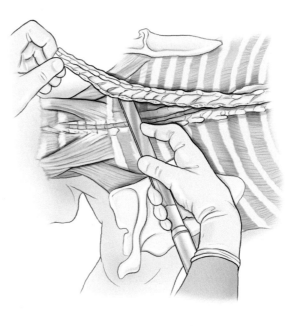

FIGURE 4-4
Laminectomy.

Remove the laminae with an osteotome or snips to expose the **epidural space** (N170; G4.49; GY47; C360, 361).

Observe the paired **ligamentum flavum** joining adjacent laminae on the deep surface. These elastic ligaments are thickest in the lumbar region where they assist with extension of the vertebral column after flexion.

Observe the dura mater (N169; G4.43, 4.49; GY49; C358). Note that the dura is not fused to the **periosteum** of the vertebral canal. Instead, a fat-filled **epidural space** is found.

Incise the dura longitudinally to expose the **conus medullaris, filum terminale,** and **cauda equina** (N160; G4.41, 4.44; GY45; C359).

Observe that the spinal cord does not extend below the level of L2 but that spinal nerves continue caudally to emerge from lower lumbar and **sacral foramina** (N161; G4.43; GY44; C357). The dural sac ends at the level of S2. The external filum terminale anchors the dural sac to the coccygeal vertebrae.

Trace a dorsal root laterally and remove any remaining bone obscuring the intervertebral foramen.

Incise the dura sac laterally and locate the dorsal root ganglion. Note that the dura mater is continuous with the epineurium of the peripheral nerve.

Identify (N169; G4.44, 4.46; GY49; C358): arachnoid mater, **pia mater, denticulate ligaments, ventral and dorsal roots,** and **spinal ganglion (dorsal root ganglion).**

Cut several spinal nerves on one side, and retract the spinal cord and dural sheath to the other side.

Clean the **posterior longitudinal ligament** (N159; G4.18; GY35). The posterior longitudinal ligament narrows considerably in the lumbar region and provides little support to the intervertebral discs here. Compare this width with the **anterior longitudinal ligament** width. Note its fusion to the annulus fibrosis of the intervertebral disc.

Exercises

1. On the figure, draw in the cell bodies of a primary sensory neuron and an alpha motor neuron, and indicate the course of their axons.

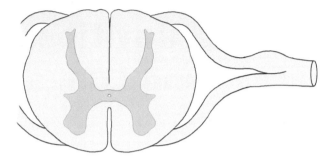

2. Why is a lumbar puncture performed at L3-L4 or L4-L5? List in order the tissues traversed by the needle.

3. What factors combine to explain the high incidence of disc herniation in the lumbar region of the vertebral column? Painful symptoms are typically experienced on only one side. Why?

4. On the figure below, indicate the cutaneous sensory distribution of the dorsal rami of spinal nerves.

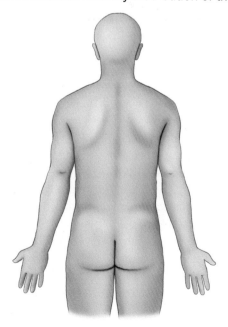

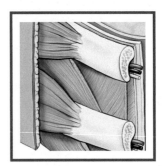

Thoracic Body Wall, Pleural Cavities, and Lungs

LAB OBJECTIVES

In this lab the musculoskeletal anatomy of the thoracic body wall will be examined and its relationship to respiration considered. The lungs will be considered in situ and then removed and examined. The extent of the pleural cavity will be explored further. On completion the student should be able to:

- Describe the development of the thoracic body wall and its mesothelial lining.
- Identify the bony landmarks of the ribs and sternum, the joints, and ligaments and how they permit or constrain movements of the ribs.
- Identify the muscles of respiration, their innervations, and actions.
- Describe the extent of the pleural cavity, its surface projections, and regional designations.
- Identify the structures associated with the hilum of the lung.
- Describe the lobar and segmental organization of the lung.

CASE STUDY

Rocky Postoperative Course

Yolanda, a 66 **y/o** woman, was in the postoperative unit at a local hospital after having undergone a total knee arthroplasty **(TKA)** 2 days ago. The surgical report indicated the procedure went well, and she was being prepared for her first bedside physical therapy visit. As a matter of course, blood pressure, heart rate, and respiration rate were taken before the therapist's visit, helping her sit at bedside, stand, and then ambulate. The therapist instructed Yolanda in the use of a rolling walker and proceeded to walk the patient with contact guard **(CG)** for 30 feet down the hallway. On the return, the patient complained of some diffuse chest pain, difficulty breathing (dyspnea), and increased breath rate (tachypnea), and she said she felt as though her heart was racing (tachycardia). The therapist assisted her back to

her room and to her bed. Vital signs were measured again and indeed all were elevated, and she indicated that she felt "anxious." She also suggested that her **R** leg felt a little tight just behind the knee. The nurse was called, and the episode was documented. Later that afternoon, Yolanda began to cough, and the nurse noticed evidence of **hemoptysis** (blood in the sputum).

Identification of the Anatomy

Identify bony structures, viscera, connective tissue, and major vessels. Also identify the components of the sternum, adjacent costochondral joints, and other bony landmarks on the anterior chest and inner chest wall.

Appreciate the following structures during dissection:

Lungs and their respective lobes
Mediastinal pleura

Bronchi and segments
Diaphragm
Internal mammary arteries
Pulmonary artery and vein
Internal and external intercostal musculature

Questions

1. What may have contributed to the signs and symptoms of this patient during her ambulation?
2. During surgery the patient is under anesthesia. How does anesthesia alter body function?
3. Any surgery conducted under general or spinal anesthesia may alter hemodynamic function and present some risks for recovery. What are common complications after surgery?

Discussion

Yolanda has some of the common signs and symptoms of a pulmonary embolism **(PE)**. Although some of these signs and symptoms may be indicative of other pulmonary compromise, they still need to be addressed because a PE may be life threatening. A **PE** is a portion of a clot or **DVT** traveling to somewhere else in the body. Some PEs are small and dissolve with the use of anticoagulant medications. Others, however, can cause immediate death if they are large enough to block both pulmonary arteries (saddle block embolus). Most commonly, the **DVT** arises from the lower extremity where blood tends to pool after surgery or stays of immobility. Lower-extremity surgeries pose a much larger risk because the surgical insult compromises soft tissue, vessels, bone, and fat, which can serve as the cause of **DVT** and give rise to an embolus. Several scales have been developed to classify the risks of developing **DVT,** and therapists should become familiar with them (i.e., Altar and Well's). Patients who have undergone surgery are almost always asked to begin motion and ambulation to increase general blood circulation through the muscle pump, heart, and lung functions. Monitoring the vital signs of patients allows the therapist to note alterations in bodily functions and help identify other possibly serious comorbidities in patients.

Preparation

Identify on the **ribs** (N185, 186; G1.9-1.11; GY57-61; C104-107):

Head
Neck
Tubercle
Angle (manubriosternal joint)
Articular facets
Costal groove
Costal cartilages
Identify on the **sternum**:
Manubrium
Angle
Body
Xiphoid process

Examine the ribcage of an articulated skeleton (N186; G1.10; GY61; C104). Note the orientation of the ribs relative to the vertebral column and to the sternum—ribs course anteriorly and inferiorly. The articulations of the head and tubercle of the rib with the body and the transverse process of the vertebra **(costovertebral joints)** form synovial (diarthritic) joints. The costal cartilages of the first ribs form as simple synchondroses with the manubrium (N186; G1.10; GY61; C104). The articulations between the costal cartilages and the sternum **(chondrosternal joints)** of ribs two through seven are secondarily synovial joints.

When the ribs are elevated, two respiratory motions can be described: **pump-handle** and **bucket-handle** motions. Estimate the axis of rotation for the ribs defined largely by their two-point articulation with the vertebrae (N187; G1.13; GY60; C346, 347). The transverse processes of the upper thoracic vertebrae are more laterally directed; thus the axis of rotation is more medial-lateral. This motion defines the pump-handle motion of the upper ribs that elevates and protracts the sternum. The transverse processes of the lower thoracic vertebrae are more posteriorly directed; thus the axis of rotation is more anteroposterior. This motion defines the bucket-handle action of the lower ribs, which increases the breadth of the lower rib cage (Figure 5-1).

Examine the articulated skeleton, and correlate the disposition of the **lobes** and **fissures** of the lung with the rib cage (N196, 197; G1.22, 1.40; GY74, 75, 119; C109, 114, 115, 116). On yourself or a lab partner, palpate the ribs, and indicate the position of the **oblique fissure** and **horizontal fissure**. *At what rib does the oblique fissure cross the **mid-axillary line**? What costal cartilage intersects the horizontal fissure of the right lung? The inferior-most extent of the lungs crosses what rib at the mid-axillary line?*

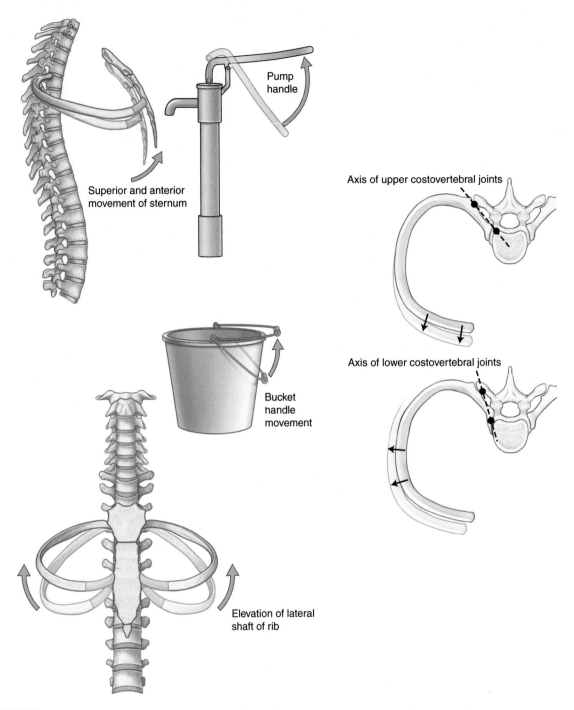

FIGURE 5-1

Movements of the thoracic wall during breathing, illustrating the so-called *pump-handle* and *bucket-handle* motions determined by the axis of rotation of the costovertebral joints. *(Modified from Drake R et al: Gray's anatomy for students, Figure 3-34, Philadelphia, 2005, Churchill Livingstone.)*

Examine a cross-section at the level of the **hilum** of the lung (**N245; GY118; C171**). Note the reflection of the parietal pleura onto the **root of the lung** to become the visceral pleura.

Anatomic Overview

Return to the trilaminar embryo. The **lateral plate mesoderm** splits into the somatic and visceral layers, creating the **intraembryonic coelom** (Figure 5-2). On lateral bending of the embryo,

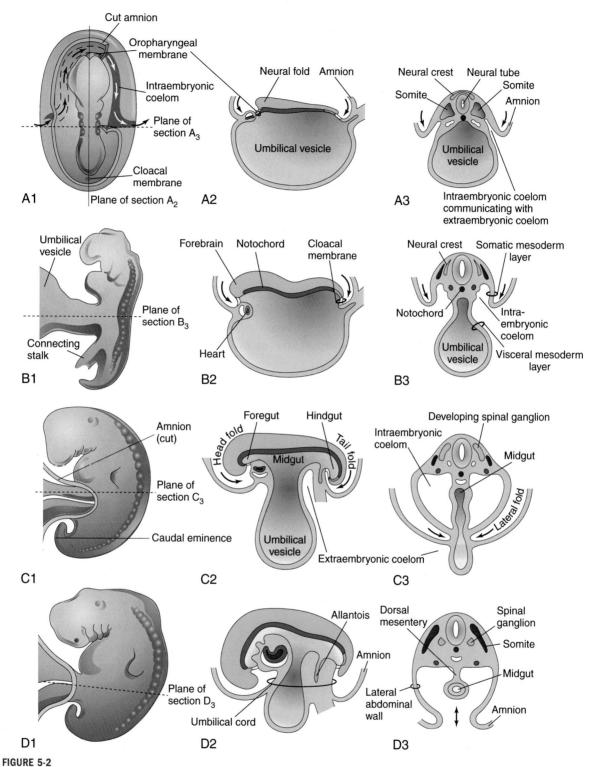

FIGURE 5-2

Lateral folding of the embryo producing the body cavity, or coelom. *(From Moore K, Persaud TVN: Before we are born: essentials of embryology and birth defects, ed 6, Philadelphia, 2008, WB Saunders.)*

the visceral layer gives rise to the smooth muscle surrounding the gastrointestinal tract; the somatic layer gives rise to the connective tissue of the body wall, excepting the ribs, which are outgrowths of the vertebrae (i.e., sclerotome), skeletal muscle, and dermis. The body wall receives migrating cells from the **hypaxial dermomyotomes,** which become the skeletal muscles, that is, intercostal and abdominal muscles, and overlying dermis. The dermomyotome cells from the hypomere bring along their innervation by ventral rami of spinal nerves. Review the anatomy of a typical spinal nerve **(N180; G1.18; GY72; C8)** and the pattern of dermatomes on the thoracic body wall **(N164; G1.6, 4.49; GY16; C8).**

The cells lining the interior of the thoracic body wall form a **serous membrane,** the **parietal pleura** (Figure 5-3). It consists of a single layer of simple squamous epithelium. Given that it derives from mesoderm, it is called a **mesothelium.**

Beneath the mesothelial cells is a basal lamina and supporting connective tissue known as the endothoracic fascia. The mesothelium secretes watery **serous fluid** that creates surface adhesion between the parietal and visceral layers of the pleura and allows the body wall and lung to slide against one another with minimal friction.

The lungs contain conducting passages, respiratory passages, and vasculature **(N204, 205).** Hyaline cartilage plates serve to maintain patency (hold them open) of the conducting passages and to reinforce the walls of the bronchi. Deeper lies a layer of spirally disposed smooth muscle and longitudinally oriented elastic fibers, the lamina propria. The elasticity of the healthy lung plays a very significant role in the mechanics of breathing. The bronchioles lack cartilage but show more prominence of the smooth muscle layer. The respiratory portion of the bronchial tree, called the **acinus,** consists of the respiratory bronchiole

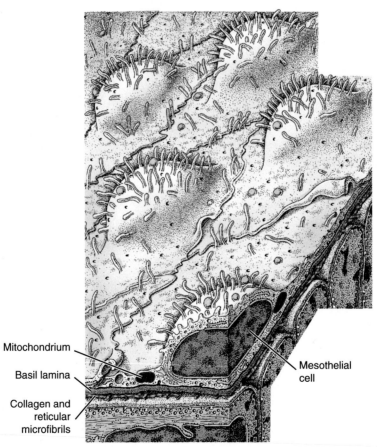

Mitochondrium

Basil lamina

Collagen and reticular microfibrils

Mesothelial cell

FIGURE 5-3

The serous membrane forming the pleura. *(Modified from Krstic RV: General histology of the mammal, Berlin, 1984, Springer-Verlag.)*

and the alveoli. This portion lacks smooth muscle. A thin layer of reticular, collagen, and elastic fibers support the epithelium.

The lungs have a dual blood supply: the pulmonary system, which conducts deoxygenated blood from the right side of the heart through the alveolar capillary beds, and the bronchial system, which arises as small branches of the aorta to supply the conducting passages of the bronchial tree and the pleura. It joins with and returns by way of the pulmonary veins.

Dissection

Place the cadaver in a supine position.

Trace the **cephalic vein** within the deltopectoral groove, and **review** the cutaneous nerves of the anterior thorax before removing the skin from the thorax (**N188; G1.2; C13**).

Make a midline incision down the length of the sternum, and then **cut** inferolaterally along the costal margins until the midaxillary line is reached.

Reflect and remove the skin flap along with the superficial fascia, taking note of examples of segmental cutaneous nerves.

Review the scheme of the typical spinal nerve (**N180, 258; G1.18; GY72; C8-7**). *What branches are encountered?*

Carefully **clean** the **pectoralis major**, and **define** its attachments (**N188; G1.2; GY64; C13**). Much of the anterior body wall is obscured by the pectoral muscles.

Cut the muscle approximately 1 cm from its sternocostal and clavicular attachments and reflect it (its innervation will be discussed later). **Observe** that the **clavipectoral fascia** is continuous with the epimysium of the **pectoralis minor** and the **subclavius** muscle (**N428; G6.18; GY64; C15**).

Cut the pectoralis minor approximately 1 cm from its attachment and **reflect** it laterally as well.

Clean away the remains of the clavipectoral fascia.

Examine the **external intercostal** muscles (**N189; G1.19; GY65, 66; C102**). The fibers run inferior and anteriorly between adjacent ribs (this is the same orientation as your fingers when placing your hands in your front pockets). The fibers end anteriorly at approximately the articulation of the ribs with the costal cartilages. The epimysium continues beyond as the external intercostal membrane.

Incise this membrane at the fourth intercostal space, just lateral to the sternum, and **insert** a probe beneath it. Using the probe as a guide, **cut** the membrane and the external intercostal muscle from the superior rib and reflect it inferiorly.

Identify the fibers of the **internal intercostal** muscle, running perpendicular to the external intercostal fibers. They extend from the angle of the rib to the most anterior limits of the intercostal spaces.

Carefully **detach** the internal intercostals from the superior rib and reflect it inferiorly. Use a blunt probe to pull down the **intercostal nerve and vessels** from the intercostals groove. Note that these neurovascular structures travel between the fibers of the internal and **innermost intercostal** muscles, or their fascias (Figure 5-4).

TIP These structures are sometimes small and difficult to locate. They can be examined further once the anterior thoracic wall has been removed.

Turn to the sternocostal joints (**N186; G1.10; GY61; C107**). **Radiate ligaments** reinforce the capsules of these synovial joints. The cavity is divided in two by the **intraarticular ligament**. With a sharp scalpel, **shave** away the anterior aspect of the joint, and expose the cavity. In some cases, fibrous union may obliterate the cavity.

Define and **partially reflect** the attachments of the **serratus anterior** from the ribs. **Review** and **preserve** the **long thoracic nerve**, which supplies this muscle.

Define the attachment of the **rectus abdominis** and **reflect** it inferiorly from its attachment to the ribs and sternum.

Using the bone, saw carefully **cut** the sternum transversely just inferior to the first rib.

Extend the cut with a scalpel along the first intercostal space, taking care to avoid cutting the deeper organs, and then inferiorly with the bone saw again along the mid-axillary line to the seventh intercostal space.

Cut along the seventh intercostal space toward the sternum, then **saw** through the xiphisternal joint.

Remove the rib cage and **examine** its deep surface, noting the shiny mesothelial membrane, the parietal pleura, lining its inner surface (**N191; G1.20; GY66; C111**). Note the innermost intercostals. Their fibers are oriented the same direction as the internal intercostals and would be nearly impossible to distinguish, except that the intercostal nerves and vessels travel between these two layers (**N192;**

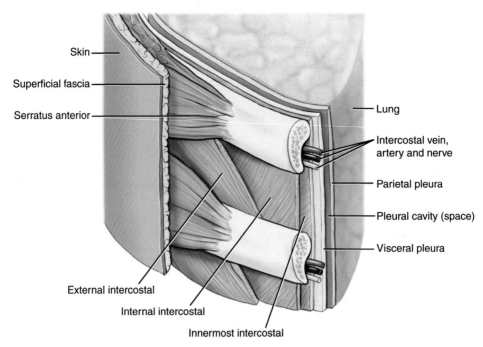

FIGURE 5-4
Cut-away of the components of the thoracic body wall.

G1.18; GY72; C158, 159). Notice where the neurovascular bundle emerges at the anterior axillary line. The **transversus thoracis** are found behind the sternum between intercostal spaces two through six. They are a continuation of the innermost intercostals layer but are oriented at right angles to the internal and innermost intercostals and are thus readily distinguished.

Identify the **internal thoracic artery**, a branch of the subclavian artery (N191; G1.20; GY66; C111). Notice the anastomoses with the intercostal arteries (N192; G1.18; GY72; C158, 159). The internal thoracic artery divides near the sixth rib into the **superior epigastric** artery and the **musculophrenic artery.**

RESPIRATORY FUNCTION OF THE INTERCOSTALS MUSCLES

Electromyographic studies have not produced uniform results regarding the intercostals' respiratory function. In general, the external intercostals and the parasternal portions of the internal intercostals are active during respiration. The remaining internal intercostals, innermost intercostals, and transversus thoracis are active as a unit during expiration.

Retract the lungs laterally, and **identify** the **root of the lung** and **pulmonary ligament** (N199, 206; G1.29, 1.30; GY76, 77; C108, 121). The ligament effectively partitions the anteroinferior region of the pleural sac from the posteroinferior.

Clinical Note

Pleuritis (Pleurisy)

Generally the serous fluid moistened layers of the pleura slide past one another during breathing; however, inflammation of the pleura causes the membranes to become rough and rub against one another. The inflammation may result from pneumonia, pulmonary infarction, or chest wall abscess. Pleuritis is characterized by dyspnea and stabbing pain, leading to restriction of ordinary breathing and spasm. Extensive inflammation results in an effusion, an accumulation of exudates in the pleural space. Fibrous adhesions may develop between the adjacent layers of the pleural membrane. Obliteration of the pleural cavity during surgery (pleurectomy) does not cause significant functional consequences; however, it may produce pain during exertion.

Cut the pulmonary vessels and the **primary bronchi,** and **cut** the pulmonary ligament. Occasionally, adhesions develop between the parietal and visceral pleura as the result of infection or inflammation.

Detach any adhesions and remove the lungs; rinse them and place them on a tray. **Wash out** the pleural sac and explore its limits. The **cupula** is the uppermost limit of the pleural sac over the apex of the lung, and it extends above the first rib into the neck (N196; G1.22; GY74; C109).

Identify the **costodiaphragmatic recesses**. The **parietal pleura** that covers the diaphragm is also called the **diaphragmatic pleura** (N194; G1.70). The diaphragm is innervated by the **phrenic nerves** (C3-5).

Locate the phrenic nerves between the mediastinal pleura and the pericardium (mesothelial sac surrounding the heart) anterior to the pulmonary vessels and bronchi (N193, 230, 231; G1.76, 1.77; GY86, 108, 110; C126, 127, 130). **Trace** them to the diaphragm.

Carefully **peel away** the **mediastinal pleura**. Note that, near the angles of the ribs, the innermost intercostals have slips that span two or more ribs and are called **subcostal** muscles (N258; G1.15; GY66).

Refer to the isolated lungs. **Identify** the **costal, medial** and **diaphragmatic (basal) surfaces** (N199, 206; G1.29, 1.30; GY76, 77; C120, 135). The **anterior** and **inferior borders** are sharp and are associated with the mediastinal and diaphragmatic recesses of the pleural sac, respectively.

Notice the **cardiac notch** on the anterior border of the left lung.

The **posterior border** is rounded and conforms to the **paravertebral gutters** (N241; G1.25, 1.78; GY73). The **apex** of the lung is blunt and conforms to the **cupula** of the pleura. The right lung is shorter than the left. It is divided into an upper and a lower lobe by an oblique fissure. A **horizontal fissure,** making a middle lobe, further divides the upper lobe. The left lung has only two lobes, presumably because of the encroachment of the heart. The embalmed lung is fixed, often preserving contact impressions of neighboring structures. Examining these impressions will help you visualize the relationship of the isolated lung to other structures in the thorax (N199, 206; G1.29, 1.30; GY76, 77; C120).

Identify the cardiac impression and the impression of the aortic arch and descending aorta on the medial surface of the left lung. On the right lung, **identify** the cardiac impression, the groove for the superior vena cava and azygous veins, and the groove for the esophagus. Impressions of the ribs may be present as well.

Examine the **hilum** of the lung (Figure 5-5). **Identify** the bronchi, pulmonary arteries, and pulmonary veins. Generally the bronchus lies centrally and posteriorly, the arteries superiorly, and the veins anteriorly and inferiorly. This relationship will vary depending on how close to the lung the root was severed. For example, in the right lung, the superior lobar branch often lies superior to the pulmonary artery. The bronchus can be readily identified by the presence of whitish cartilaginous plates, both visible and palpable.

Identify the **main** or **primary bronchus** if present. If the cut was made very close to the lung, the primary bronchus may be attached to the trachea.

Find the **secondary** or **lobar bronchi** (also known as *division* branches). In the right lung, **identify** a superior and intermediate bronchus. The intermediate bronchus eventually divides into a middle and inferior within the substance of the lung (N202, 203; G1.31; GY80, 81; C122). The left lung has a superior and an inferior lobar bronchus.

Follow the **tertiary** or **segmental bronchi**. The **bronchopulmonary segments** are the functional subunits of the lobes. They are separated from one another by connective tissue septa that are continuous with the visceral pleura. Pulmonary disorders may be localized with a bronchopulmonary segment, and surgically resecting a single segment is feasible. The branches of the pulmonary arteries accompany the bronchi, and each segment tends to have its own unique blood supply. The pulmonary veins return along the **intersegmental septa** (N205).

Using blunt dissection and the scissor technique, **clean away** the lung tissue from the hilum, and **trace** the bronchial tree to the segmental level (N199; G1.33, 1.34; C117). The pulmonary arteries carry deoxygenated blood away from the heart under pressure to overcome the resistance of the pulmonary capillary bed. Thus the artery walls are thicker and hold their cross-sectional shape. The pulmonary veins are under low pressure, and therefore their walls are much thinner. **Examine** the surface projections of the segments of the lung depicted schematically (N200, 201; G1.31; GY81; C121).

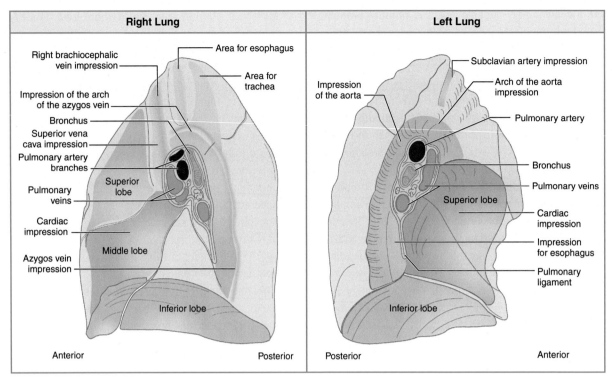

FIGURE 5-5

Sagittal section of structures located at the hilum of the lung. *(From Bogart B, Ort V:* Elsevier's integrated anatomy and embryology, *Philadelphia, 2007, WB Saunders.)*

Using a long sectioning knife, **cut** several horizontal sections completely through the inferior lobe of the right lung several centimeters above the base. These cuts should intersect the boundaries between the four basal segments of the inferior lobe. Attempt to **identify** the segmental bronchi, the pulmonary arteries, and pulmonary veins.

Exercises

1. Besides the intercostals, what other muscles act on the ribcage and thereby might influence thoracic volume during respiration (i.e., function as *accessory muscles of respiration*)?

2. On the figure, draw in and label the ligaments that support the head, neck, and angle of the ribs at the costovertebral articulations.

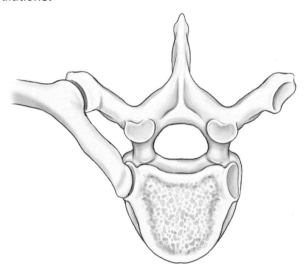

3. What dermatome corresponds with the clavicle, male nipple line, and xyphoid process?

4. What effect on respiration has reduced motion in the costovertebral joints?

5. While referring to your atlas, examine the tracing of a lateral radiograph of the lungs, and label below as many of the segmental bronchi as possible.

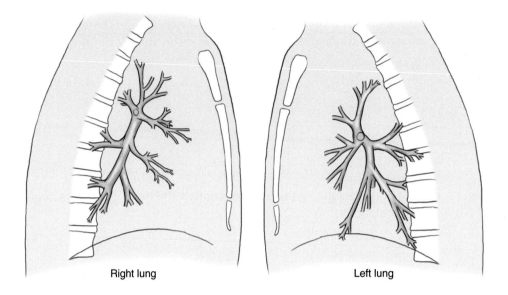

Right lung   Left lung

6. On the figure, color in and label the surface projections of the bronchopulmonary segments. Note the distinctions between right and left lungs.

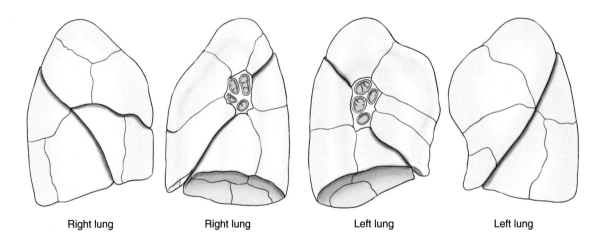

Right lung   Right lung   Left lung   Left lung

7. What would the postural drainage position be for patients with infiltrates in the various segments of their lungs? Think gravity!

Heart and Mediastinum

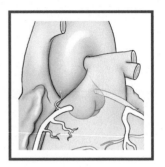

LAB OBJECTIVES

In this lab the student will observe the heart and its coverings *in situ* and its relationship to structures within the mediastinum. The heart will then be removed for a closer examination of its internal anatomy and vasculature. On completion the student should be able to:

- Describe the development of the heart and histology of cardiac muscle.
- Identify the pericardium and its parts.
- Trace the flow of blood through the heart, describing chambers, valves, major vessels, and coronary circulation.
- Identify the major branches and tributaries of the great vessels of the heart.
- Define the boundaries and contents of the mediastinum.

CASE STUDY

Heart Attack or Heartburn?

A 45 **y/o** male engineer is seen in the **ER** and **c/o** intense mid-scapular pain, shoulder pain, and minor substernal pain. He indicates to the physician that he was working on his garage last evening putting up insulation and then began having pain this morning after breakfast. He tried to lie down, but this action increased the pain. The patient thought the pain was a muscle ache, given that he was not used to doing hard labor, and he wanted to just make sure it was not anything serious. He further indicates that he felt some pain below the sternum and the right side of the neck and felt as though he was having a "heart attack" after breakfast. His **PMH** is mostly unremarkable other than having some similar symptoms over the previous year when he eats too much, especially when he is "on the go." The physician conducts a general upper quarter screen **(UQS),** which is unremarkable other than the upper back pain became stronger when the patient was asked to lean forward at the waist, inhale deeply or rotate the torso to the **R** or **L.** Vital signs **(VS)** were normal, with **BP** 124/86 mm Hg, **HR** 70 beats per minute, and **RR** 12 breaths per minute. The physician conducts an **ECG** with the patient supine, and the findings are normal. The physician suggests that the patient see a physical therapist because she believs the pain was musculoskeletal in nature. A prescription of ibuprofen is given, and the patient is told to come back in 2 weeks if the symptoms did not subside after therapy for his muscle spasms.

Identification of the Anatomy

The thorax houses numerous vital organs and is separated into various regions. The mediastinum within the thoracic cavity contains the heart. The lungs are clearly visible to the right and left of the mediastinum and the diaphragm is located inferior to the heart. An appreciation of the viscera in the posterior mediastinum is important because the major blood vessels and other structures in this area dive inferiorly through the diaphragm and follow the anterior aspect of the vertebral column.

Appreciate the following structures during dissection:

- Bony thorax, including ribs, sternum (sternal notch and angle of Louie), xiphoid process, sternoclavicular joints and sternocostal borders
- Trachea
- Esophagus and cardiac sphincter
- Descending aorta
- Inferior and superior vena cava
- Diaphragm with central tendon and left and right hemi-diaphragm
- Fibrous mediastinum with all divisions

Questions

1. Given the visualized anatomy in your dissection, what other structures in the thoracic cavity and mediastinum may contribute to this patient's signs and symptoms?
2. The postural change bringing on this patient's symptoms may be related to the possibility of what structure in the thoracic cavity being compromised?
3. What is the cause of the upper back pain?

Discussion

Although a patient's signs and symptoms may lead a clinician to believe the problem to be musculoskeletal in origin, sometimes this diagnosis is far from accurate. The thoracic cavity with its contents can be disrupted by several problems that may *refer* pain and discomfort to regions away from the true site of the pathologic condition. In this case a condition known as gastroesophageal reflux disease **(GERD)** is probably the case, but it would have to be further diagnosed with radiographs, esophageal manometry, and esophagoscopy; pH monitoring would further define the diagnosis. The classic symptom of this problem is regurgitation and heartburn especially after large meals. It is the result of the incompetence of the lower esophageal sphincter, which allows gastric acids to move into the lower esophagus from the stomach. The patient's increase in the symptoms when changing postures or deep breathing allowed for the movement of gastric contents to *reflux* into the esophagus. In turn, the nerves in this area sometimes refer the symptoms such as pain or tightness to the upper back, neck, sternum or shoulder, hence the erroneous

inference of musculoskeletal problems. **GERD** is a serious condition that may cause esophageal stricture, ulcer, hemorrhage, and cell changes leading to carcinoma. This patient should be referred back to the primary physician for further study.

Preparation

On the articulated skeleton, note the anterior projection of the heart. It lies deep to the **body of the sternum (N196; G1.40; GY85; C109, 129)**. The **superior border (base)** of the heart coincides roughly with the **sternal angle,** or slightly below it. The **right border** of the heart is formed by the right atrium and lies approximately one finger's breadth (fb) lateral to the sternum. The **inferior border** is formed largely by the right ventricle and roughly coincides with the **xiphisternal joint.** Here the heart lies on the central tendon of the diaphragm. The inferior border extends one hand's breadth to the left of the sternum, ending at the **apex,** in the fifth intercostal space, medial to the **midclavicular line.** The **left border** corresponds to the left ventricle and proceeds from the apex to a point one fb lateral to the sternum at the second costal cartilage.

Anatomic Overview

The heart begins development at the cranial end of the embryonic disc, in the visceral (splanchnic) portion of the **lateral plate mesoderm** (Figure 6-1). During cephalic and lateral folding, the paired **heart tubes** are brought together ventral to the foregut. They undergo a complex process of folding and remodeling, eventually resulting in four chambers. The heart tubes are accompanied by the **pericardial coelom,** into which the heart sinks.

The **pericardial sac** is lined by a mesothelium with a visceral and parietal layer. The visceral layer together with a variable thickness of fat is called the **epicardium.** The parietal layer becomes surrounded by fibrous connective tissue and becomes the **pericardium.** The mesenchyme surrounding the heart tubes proliferates and differentiates to become the **myocardium.** Cardiac muscle is distinguished from skeletal muscle in several ways (Figure 6-2). The cells have a single, centrally placed nucleus; branch, bifurcate, and anastomose freely; are joined by intercalated discs; and possess a capillary-rich endomysium.

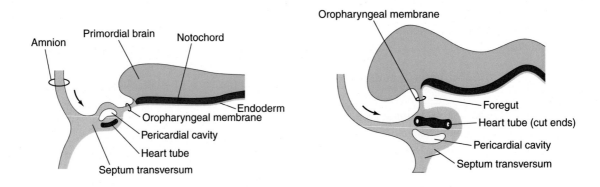

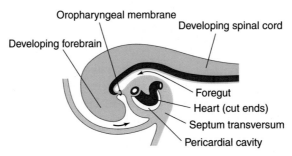

FIGURE 6-1

Early development of the heart. *(From Moore K, Persaud TVN: Before we are born: essentials of embryology and birth defects, ed 7, Philadelphia, 2008, WB Saunders.)*

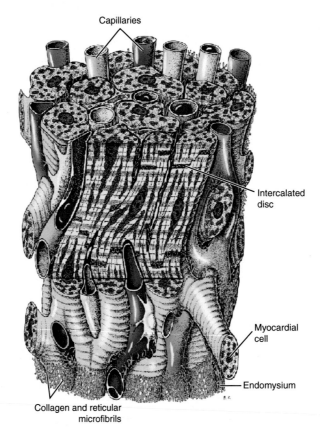

FIGURE 6-2

Histology of myocardial tissue. *(Modified from Krstic RV: General histology of the mammal, Berlin, 1984, Springer-Verlag.)*

The heart is located within the **mediastinum** (N230, 231, 241; G1.25, 1.75, 1.76; GY85, 108, 110; C126, 127). The mediastinum is that part of the thoracic cavity between the two pleural sacs. It contains all the thoracic viscera except the lungs and is encompassed by an extension of the thoracic subserous fascia. The mediastinum is arbitrarily divided into four regions. The **superior mediastinum** lies above a horizontal plane running through the sternal angle and the intervertebral disc 4/5. This plane also coincides with the upper limit of the fibrous pericardium and level of the bifurcation of the trachea. The **anterior mediastinum** is the potential space between the sternum and the pericardium; the **middle mediastinum** contains the pericardial sac and the heart; the **posterior mediastinum** extends to the vertebral column. *Name the major structures located in the posterior mediastinum.*

Clinical Note

Subdivisions of the mediastinum

Radiographic conventions differ slightly in the designations of the regions of the mediastinum. The anterior mediastinum extends from the sternum to the back of the pericardial sac; the middle mediastinum extends from the pericardium to a line approximately 1 cm back from the anterior margin of the vertebral column; the posterior comprises the paravertebral spaces. The term superior mediastinum is deleted.

Dissection

Examine the pericardium surrounding the heart *in situ* (N211; G1.21; GY86; C130).

Locate the **phrenic nerve**. **Notice** that it courses between the pericardium and mediastinal pleura, anterior to the pulmonary vessels, on its way to the diaphragm.

Nick the pericardium in the midline near the base of the heart. Using scissors, **make** a vertical cut carried to the inferior border, then **extend** the cut to the right and left along the inferior border. Rinse out the interior of the pericardial sac. Contrast the smooth shiny inner surface **(serous layer)** to the outer dull coarse **fibrous** layer of the pericardial sac.

Place your fingers in the **transverse pericardial sinus** (N215; G1.44; GY87; C134, 135).

Using scissors, **cut** the ascending **aorta** and the **pulmonary trunk** just below their pericardial reflections.

Cut the **superior vena cava** and **inferior vena cava** just within their reflections of pericardium.

Lift the heart upward and cut the four **pulmonary veins.** All that is holding the heart in place is the double layer of pericardium separating the transverse pericardial sinus from the **oblique pericardial sinus. Cut** it with a scalpel and remove the heart. Orientation of the isolated heart can be a challenge initially.

Identify the **superior** and **inferior vena cava,** which empty in the right atrium. **Pass** a single probe through these vessels. In anatomic position, the probe should be vertically oriented and lie just posterior to the right border of the heart as seen in anterior view.

Examine the exterior of the heart (N214; G1.41; GY88, 89; C132, 133, 137).

Identify the eight **great vessels:**

Superior vena cava
Inferior vena cava
Aorta
Pulmonary trunk
Pulmonary veins (4)

Trace the **coronary circulation** (N216; G1.45, 1.46; GY96; C138). Use blunt dissection to trace the coronary vessels, which lie beneath the epicardium. A significant amount of fat may be found between the epicardium and myocardium. Note common variations (N217; G148; GY97, 98; C139).

Unless instructed otherwise, **make** the incisions depicted in Figure 6-3.

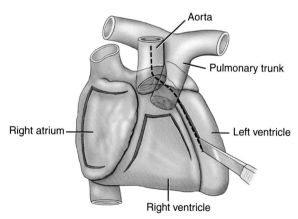

FIGURE 6-3
Incisions exposing the chambers of the heart.

Clean out any clotted blood and rinse out the chambers of the heart.

Examine the interior of the chambers, and **identify** the following structures (N220, 221; G1.49-1.52; GY99; C129-135):

Right atrium
  Right auricle
  Pectinate muscles
  Crista terminalis
  Fossa ovalis
  Coronary sinus
  Valve of inferior vena cava
  Tricuspid valve
Right ventricle
  Tricuspid valve
  Chordae tendinae
  Papillary muscles
  Trabeculae carnae
  Pulmonary semilunar valve
Left atrium
  Left auricle
  Fossa ovalis
  Bicuspid (mitral) valve
Left ventricle
  Bicuspid (mitral) valve
  Aortic semilunar valve
  Orifices of coronary arteries

Review the flow of the blood through the heart and the pulmonary and systemic circuits.

POSTERIOR MEDIASTINUM
(N230, 231; G1.76, 1.77; GY108, 110; C126, 127)

Incise the posterior aspect of the parietal pericardium and expose the posterior mediastinum (N232; G1.54, 1.59; GY106).

Notice that the **descending aorta** lies to the left of the vertebral bodies. Note also that, in addition to the intercostal arteries to the thoracic body wall, aortic branches supply the bronchi (N207; G1.72; C156) and the esophagus (N237; G1.72; C156).

Notice the left **vagus nerve** (cranial nerve X) as it leaves the descending aorta and joins the right to form the **esophageal plexus** (N240; G1.76; GY112; C152). The **esophagus** generally lies anterior to the vertebral bodies but penetrates the diaphragm just left of the midline (N233). Hence the **inferior esophageal sphincter** lies between the heart and descending aorta.

Identify the cut ends of the inferior and superior vena cava. The blood from the thoracic body wall does not return directly to the vena cava but instead drains into the **azygous** and **hemiazygous** and **accessory hemiazygous veins** located in the posterior thoracic wall (N238; G.1.75; GY113; C162). The **thoracic duct** returns lymph to the venous system via the left subclavian vein (N239; G1.73; GY113; C168).

Note the **sympathetic chain ganglia** seen lying on either side of the vertebral bodies (N209; G1.76, 1.77; GY113; C166, 167). Clean the pleural and the sympathetic chain can be seen, showing through the membrane.

Peel away the pleura on the right side, and **examine** the **sympathetic cardiac nerves** and **sympathetic pulmonary nerves.** These structures are postganglionic axons from T1-5. These nerves often join with parasympathetic nerves to form plexi at or near the target viscera (N226, 227, 240; G1.79; GY113, C166) (Figure 6-4).

Find the greater splanchnic nerve, which carries preganglionic axons to the celiac ganglion on the abdominal aorta.

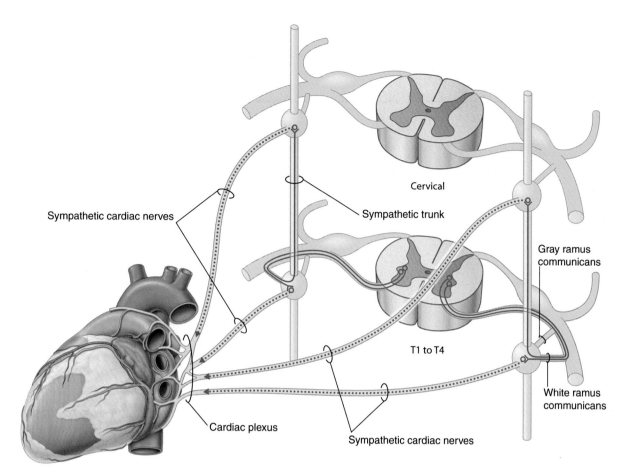

FIGURE 6-4
Path of sympathetic nerves traveling to the heart. *(From Drake R et al:* Gray's anatomy for students, *Philadelphia, 2005, Churchill Livingstone.)*

Exercises

1. Review and indicate the surface projection of the heart on the anterior bony thorax.

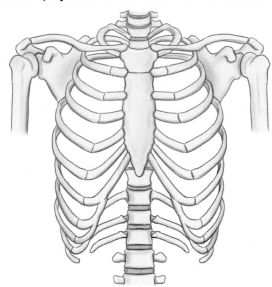

2. Correctly label the coronary vessels. Does your heart present any variation from these textbook depictions? Describe them.

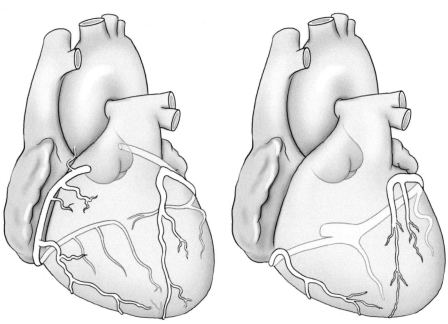

3. On the magnetic resonance image (MRI) below, identify the right and left ventricles as seen in axial section. Can you account for the difference in thickness of the respective ventricular myocardium?

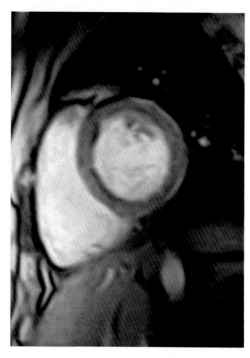

(From Kelley L, Petersen C: *Sectional anatomy for imaging professionals,* St Louis, 1997, Mosby.)

4. The topographic positions of the structures within the mediastinum can be better appreciated when considered in cross-section. Label the following structures within the superior mediastinum: trachea, esophagus, thoracic duct, brachiocephalic veins, brachiocephalic artery, left common carotid artery, vagus nerves, phrenic nerves, and sympathetic chain.

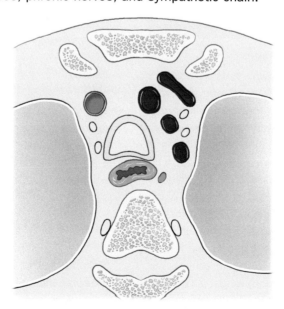

5. Describe the path of the cardiac sympathetic nerves.

LAB EXPLORATION 7

Abdominal Body Wall and Inguinal Region

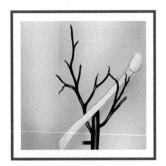

LAB OBJECTIVES

In this exploration the components of the anterior abdominal body wall will be differentiated and their relationship to the inguinal canal defined. On completion of this lab the student will be able to:

- Describe the development of the abdominal body wall and the peritoneal cavity.
- Identify the trilaminar abdominal muscles and fascia.
- Define the inguinal canal, and describe the descent of the testes.
- Discuss inguinal hernias (direct and indirect).
- Define the boundaries and contents of the femoral canal and appearance of femoral hernias.

CASE STUDY

Postpartum Abdominal Weakness

Shannon is a 35 **y/o** patient who gave birth to her first child 1 month ago and has been referred to the clinic by a clinical psychologist for evaluation of posture, nursing positioning, and abdominal strengthening. The subjective aspect of this client includes a **PMH** indicating her pregnancy was normal term; she gained approximately 20 kg and had a Caesarean delivery (C-section). She is being treated for depression and has concerns about her lack of sleep, breast pain, and shoulder pain. She also expresses being unhappy about her lack of ability to begin exercise and fitness activities such as running and skiing to achieve her pregravid body weight. She currently weighs 70 kg, with a **BMI** of 29, and indicates a loss of 5 kg since giving birth. Her C-section incision is healing nicely and measures 9 inches. It is tender to the touch. She **c/o** weak abdominals and what appears to be a severe depression in the midline of her abdominal muscles that is especially visible when she contracts them.

Identification of the Anatomy

During this dissection, you need to identify the linea alba first and then progress your dissection bilaterally to identify the various layers of the abdominal wall. The abdominal muscles may be very thin on certain specimens; thus proceed with caution during your scalpel and blunt dissections.

Appreciate the following structures during dissection:

Skin, fat, fascia, muscle
External and internal abdominal obliques
Transverse abdominis
Linea alba
Rectus sheath
Inguinal ligaments

Questions

1. Postpartum discomfort and emotional distress are not uncommon. What are some of the other signs and symptoms seen in women who have just given birth?
2. What musculature of the abdomen is altered during the pregnancy process, especially during the last trimester?
3. Can you suggest treatment interventions for this patient?

Discussion

The condition of pregnancy and birthing involve major hormonal and physical changes during the 9-month period. Women often experience emotional and physical distress symptoms long after the birth (puerperium) of a baby. Depending on the progression of the pregnancy and type of delivery, women may have depression, perineum pain, pelvic pain, weakness, hemorrhoids, constipation, mastitis, and general decrease in muscle and bladder tone. The condition of the abdominal musculature described in this patient is called **diastasis recti.** This condition is caused by the distention of the abdominal muscle during pregnancy, leading to muscle and connective-tissue separation and stretching of the rectus abdominis muscle to the point beyond its normal length. The separation may be as wide as or wider than 2 cm and will need to be strengthened to resume its normal position. Specific members of the rehabilitation team, including occupational and physical therapists, nurses, and mental health professionals, can address a wide range of interventions, including progressive exercise for the pelvic and abdominal muscles and muscles of the upper back and postural muscles, as well as posture, depression, positioning for feeding, handling the neonate, sexual activity, and weight loss.

Preparation

Identify the following skeletal landmarks (N240):

Xiphisternal joint
Costal margin
Pubic symphysis
Pubic crest
Anterior superior iliac spine
Iliac crest

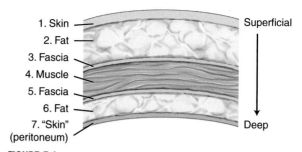

1. Skin — Superficial
2. Fat
3. Fascia
4. Muscle
5. Fascia
6. Fat
7. "Skin" (peritoneum) — Deep

FIGURE 7-1
Layers of abdominal body wall.

The abdominal cavity is enclosed anteriorly and laterally by the abdominal body wall, which is composed of several layers. These layers are the same as those comprising the thoracic body wall, except for the addition of a layer of fat of variable thickness, just superficial to the peritoneum, called the **extraperitoneal fat** (N252; G2.6; GY131; C184, 186) (Figure 7-1). In addition, you will see a membrane, the **transversalis fascia,** described as a continuation of the epimysium of the **transversus abdominis,** but considered by others to be a part of the extraperitoneal connective tissue.

Anatomic Overview

Return to the trilaminar embryo. You will recall that the **lateral plate mesoderm** splits into the **parietal (somatic)** and **visceral (splancnic)** layers, creating the **intraembryonic coelom.** On lateral folding of the embryo, the visceral layer gives rise to the smooth muscle surrounding the gastrointestinal tract—the parietal layer to the connective tissue of the body wall (except the skeletal muscles). The abdominal body wall receives migrating cells from the **hypaxial dermomyotomes,** which become the abdominal muscles, and overlying dermis in this region. The dermomyotome cells from the hypomere receive their sensory and motor innervation by ventral rami of spinal nerves. Review the anatomic features of a typical spinal nerve (N180, 258; G1.18; GY72; C8).

The cells lining the interior of the abdominal body cavity form a **serous membrane,** the **peritoneum.** It consists of a single layer of simple squamous epithelium. Because it derives from mesenchyme from the mesoderm, it is traditionally called the **mesothelium.** Beneath the mesothelial cells is a basal lamina and supporting connective tissue. The mesothelium secretes a watery **serous fluid,** which forms a film of fluid filling the potential space of the peritoneal cavity, and separates **parietal peritoneum** lining the body wall from the **visceral peritoneum** covering most of the abdominal organs. The parietal and visceral peritoneum forms a continuous closed **peritoneal sac.**

We might expect that the muscles of the abdominal body wall would derive from the hypaxial myotomes of the adjacent lumbar region. However, almost all of the cells of the hypaxial dermomyotomes L2 through S3 are drawn into the formation of the pelvic limb musculature, leaving only L1 and small parts of L2 through L4 to contribute to the abdominal wall. The remainder consists largely of a trilaminar muscle block, which is homologous to the intercostal muscles, derived from hypaxial dermomyotomes T7 through L1, and the **rectus abdominis** (T7-T12). Upright posture of the trunk on extended hips subject the inguinal region to stress of intraabdominal pressure.

Dissection

Continue a midline incision to the pubic symphysis, encircling the umbilicus along the way. **Make** transverse cuts as convenient.

Skin the anterior part of the thigh to just a few centimeters below the inguinal ligament. **Remove** the skin flaps.

Attempt to **locate** the anterior cutaneous nerves of the abdominal wall (N257; G2.5; GY134; C176). The spinal nerve inferior to the twelfth rib is named the **subcostal nerve** (T12). The last nerve on the anterior of the abdomen is the **iliohypogastric nerve** (L1) running along the inguinal ligament. Note that the origin of the **external abdominal oblique** lies above the costal margin and interdigitates with slips of the serratus anterior.

Clean the surface of the external abdominal oblique, noting the anterior branches of the lateral cutaneous nerves. The **aponeurosis of the external abdominal oblique** encompasses the rectus abdominis before entwining with its contralateral half at the midline to form the **linea alba** (L. *white line,* owing to the density of collagen fibers) (N250; G2.5; GY128; C184).

The free inferior border of the aponeurosis of the external abdominal oblique muscle forms the **inguinal ligament.** It spans between the anterior-superior iliac spine and the pubic tubercle forming the **lateral crus** of the **superficial inguinal ring.** The **medial crus** passes medial to the spermatic cord in men (or round ligament of the ovary in women) and attaches to the pubic crest (N249; G2.7, 2.8; GY128; C179). The two crura are bound by **intercrural fibers.**

Split the muscle fibers of the external abdominal oblique, beginning approximately 5 cm above the iliac crest, separating them along their line of fiber orientation. **Observe** that the underlying fibers of the **internal abdominal oblique** run perpendicular to those of the external abdominal oblique (N250; G2.5; GY130; C181).

Separate the external abdominal oblique from the **internal abdominal oblique** by inserting a finger into the fascial plane between these two muscle bellies. Move your finger toward the midline until the **rectus sheath** is encountered.

Incise the aponeurosis of the external abdominal oblique 1 cm lateral to the **rectus abdominis,** and **reflect** the external abdominal oblique laterally. Leave the inguinal region intact.

Note the **ilioinguinal nerve** (L1) that emerges through the superficial ring just lateral to the spermatic cord (or round ligament of the uterus in women). It provides cutaneous innervation to the external genitals and the medial thigh. The inferior fibers of the internal abdominal oblique arc above the medial half of the inguinal ligament, creating a **submuscular gap,** a potential weak point in the anterior abdominal wall. The inguinal canal pierces the inferior margin of the internal abdominal oblique midway along the inguinal ligament, forming the **"middle"** inguinal ring.

Follow the ilioinguinal nerve proximally to the point where it pierces the internal abdominal oblique and travels between the internal abdominal oblique and the **transversus abdominis.** If possible, **insert** a finger into this intermuscular plane and pass it inferiorly, separating the inferior borders of these two muscles. If they are fused together, separation may not be possible. The combined aponeuroses join to form the **conjoint tendon (falx inguinalis)** (N259; G2.9, 2.10; GY130; C181).

Hold the free lower margin of the transversus abdominis forward and upward. **Sweep** a scalpel handle between it and underlying **transversalis fascia** (**N260; G2.14; GY138; C186**). This fascia is the internal investing fascia that lines the entire muscular abdominal wall. Deep to it a layer of **extraperitoneal fat** is found.

Turn to the rectus abdominis, and incise the sheath vertically down the middle of each muscle belly. **Detach** and **reflect** the muscles inferiorly.

> **TIP** The intersegmental tendons of the rectus abdominis, which give the six-pack appearance to the muscle belly, are attached to the sheath and must be cut to reflect the sheath and the muscle.

Examine the posterior wall of the sheath. **Identify** the **arcuate line** midway between the symphysis and umbilicus (**N251; G2.5; GY130; C177, 184**). Below the arcuate line, all aponeurotic layers pass in front of (ventral to) the rectus abdominis. Above the arcuate line, the aponeurosis of the internal abdominal oblique splits to encompass the rectus abdominis anteriorly and posteriorly (**N252; G2.6; GY131; C186**).

Inferior to the arcuate line, **insert** a probe beneath the **transversalis fascia**, separated by the **extraperitoneal fat** from the **peritoneum**, a serous membrane that lines the abdominopelvic cavity (**N253; G2.18; GY141; C186**).

Incise the linea alba along the midline, and cut the abdominal walls along the costal margins.

Review the inguinal canal and its walls (**N260; G2.14; GY138; C192**). **Gently push** a probe obliquely into the superficial inguinal ring along the spermatic cord.

Place a hand inside the peritoneal cavity, and **feel** where it pushes against the **deep inguinal ring** in the transversalis fascia. Note the continuity of the layers of the abdominal wall with the layers of the spermatic cord (Figure 7-3).

Review the relationships of the inguinal rings:

Deep inguinal ring—through the transversalis fascia and submuscular gap of the transverses abdominis

"Middle" inguinal ring—through the margin of the internal abdominal oblique

Superficial inguinal ring—through the aponeurosis of the external abdominaloblique

Remove the skin inferior to the inguinal ligament, leaving the superficial fascia in place.

Find the **great saphenous vein,** and **follow** it proximally to where it passes through the **saphenous opening,** a gap in the deep fascia of the thigh, to reach the **femoral vein** (**N249; G5.15, 5.16; GY344; C369**). The femoral vein, together with the **femoral artery** and a cluster of **lymphatics,** are encompassed by connective tissue forming the **femoral sheath** (**N262; G5.15, 5.16; GY290; C369**).

Clean away the superficial fascia. The **femoral nerve** emerges from beneath the inguinal ligament lateral to the femoral sheath and over the iliopsoas muscle.

The **inguinal ligament,** the **sartorius muscle,** and the **adductor longus muscle** bind the **femoral triangle.** The gap under the inguinal ligament is another potential location of hernias, in this case termed a **femoral hernia.** A loop of bowel insinuates under the ligament.

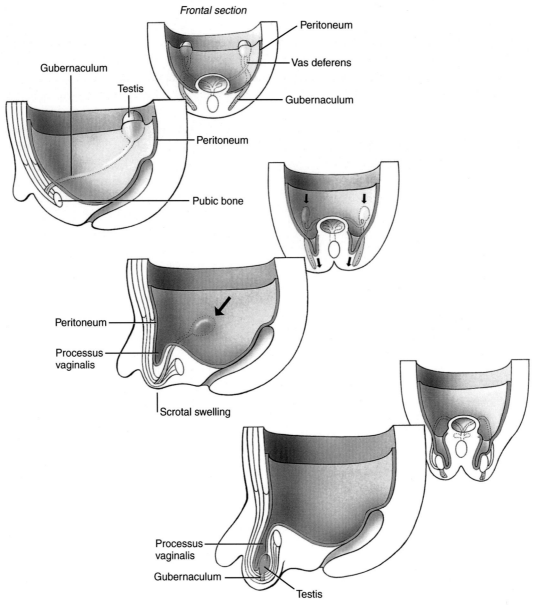

FIGURE 7-2
Pathways of the indirect and direct inguinal hernias. *(From Larsen W:* Human embryology, *ed 3, Philadelphia, 2001, Churchill Livingstone).*

Clinical Note

Turn your head and cough

The architecture of the lower abdominal region makes it a potential weak point in the body wall. In men particularly, the descent of the testicle (Figure 7-2) and spermatic cord through the inguinal canal into the scrotum may leave the patient susceptible to inguinal hernias. As the testicle is drawn into the scrotum, it brings along an outpouching of the perineum, called the processus vaginalis (Figure 7-3). If the processus vaginalis fails to obliterate properly, a loop of bowel may become insinuated through the deep inguinal ring into the inguinal canal or on into the scrotum. This condition is known as an indirect inguinal hernia. A direct inguinal hernia presses directly toward the superficial inguinal ring. The inferior epigastric artery serves as a landmark to distinguish direct from indirect hernias. A protrusion medial to the artery indicates a direct hernia; a protrusion lateral to the artery is an indirect hernia. The physician can test for patency of the inguinal canal by pressing a finger through the superficial ring against the deep ring and asking the patient to cough. The increased intraabdominal pressure accompanying the cough can be felt pushing against the examiner's finger. Similarly, increased intraabdominal pressure accompanying heavy lifting may result in an inguinal hernia.

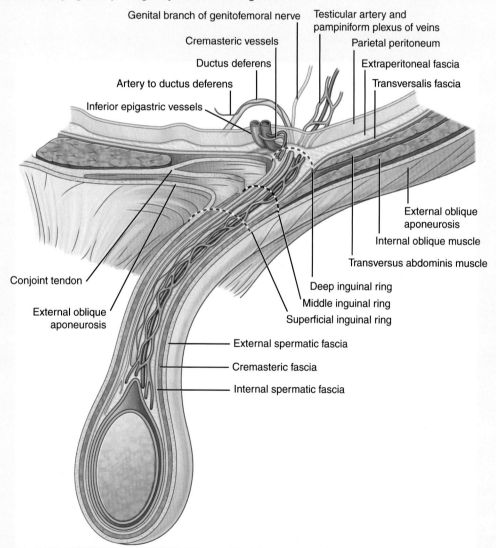

FIGURE 7-3

Observe on the left an indirect hernia, which protrudes through the deep inguinal rings lateral to the inferior epigastric vessels. On the right, notice the direct hernia protruding through the superficial ring medial to the inferior epigastric vessels. *(From Drake R et al:* Gray's anatomy for students, *Philadelphia, 2005, Churchill Livingstone.)*

Exercises

1. Describe the anatomic basis for a lower incidence of inguinal hernias in women but a higher incidence of femoral hernias in women.

2. Indicate on the figure below the relative positions of a direct and an indirect inguinal hernia.

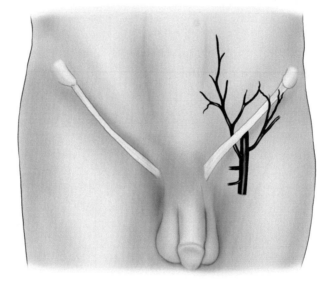

3. One might expect the anterior abdominal muscles to be innervated by lumbar spinal nerves, but this is generally not the case. Why?

4. What dermatome correlates with the umbilicus? The inguinal ligament?

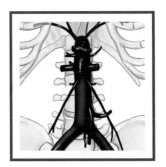

Peritoneal Cavity and Abdominal Viscera

LAB OBJECTIVES

In this lab the mesothelial lining of the abdominopelvic cavity is considered and its relationship to the gastrointestinal tract and ancillary organs. On completion of this lab the student will be able to:

- Discuss the development of the primitive gut tube and its smooth muscle.
- Describe the layers of the peritoneum, its reflections, mesenteries, ligaments, and omentae.
- Identify the ancillary organs of the GI tract.
- Identify the major branches of the abdominal aorta and tributaries of the hepatic portal vein.
- Identify the pelvic organs lying inferior to the peritoneum.

CASE STUDY

Groin Pain

Franz is a 68 **y/o** male patient referred to your **OT** clinic by family practitioner (FP) with a **cc** of **R** groin pain and difficulty tying his shoes. He states that he has experienced the pain "on and off" for sometime but recently noticed it more when he goes on his normal walks and during some of his **ADL.** He was also shoveling snow recently, and the pain increased slightly, but he attributed the episode to a pulled muscle. He also states that he is plagued with some nagging **LBP** but attributes it to his age and general deconditioning. His **PMH** and **systems review** suggest minor **LBP** and **HTN,** which he has tried to control with medications; he also has a family history of heart disease. Franz further suggests the discomfort gets a bit worse after meals and sometimes during bowel movements. He further states that sometimes he can "feel" his abdomen pulsating when lying in bed. His **LE** functional muscular strengths, sensation, **DTRs,** and dermatomal

examination are normal for his age. His active **AROM** is essential normal in both **LEs**, with slight pain in the groin and lower **R** quadrant in **R** thigh abduction. The pain does not appear to be musculature.

Identification of the Anatomy

The dissection should expose the major muscles and vessels of the peritoneal cavity. These muscles and vessels should be easily identifiable secondary to their size and strategic locations in the cavity. Take special note to identify the vessels to each organ. These factors become important in identifying the location and cause of much of his condition.

Appreciate the following structures during dissection:

Bony, muscle, and organ structures:

Anterior aspects of the lumbar vertebra, sacrum, iliac crests, kidneys, bladder, ureters, iliacus muscle, psoas muscle, and quadratus lumborum muscle

Vessels
- **Abdominal aorta**
- **Celiac artery**
- **Superior and inferior mesenteric arteries**
- **Renal arteries**
- **Common iliac arteries**
- **External and internal iliac arteries**
- **Inferior vena cava**
- **Hepatic veins**
- **Renal veins**
- **Common iliac veins**
- **External and internal iliac veins**

Questions

1. The patient experiences increased symptoms after activity, body posture, and eating. Can you postulate what may be the causing this association?
2. Referred pain is an issue in this patient. What types of conditions refer pain to the low back?
3. What is the relationship of the gait abnormality to the disease of the spine?

Discussion

At times, patients exhibit a set of signs and symptoms that may appear as though they are musculoskeletal in nature but indicate something totally different. Such is the case with Franz, who has some of the classic signs and symptoms of an abdominal aortic aneurysm **(AAA),** which is an enlargement of the abdominal aorta secondary to the degenerative process and a suggested genetic disposition. Aortic aneurysms may also occur in the aortic arch or the thoracic region. An AAA (triple A) is not that uncommon and may be initially detected by an astute health care professional through taking a complete history and general systems review. Triple A is approximately five times more prevalent in men than in woman. The onset of the problems is approximately age 50 in men and age 60 in women. Some of the classic symptoms are groin and back pain, which is referred from the enlargement of the aorta in the abdominal cavity. Prostate cancer and other diseases also refer pain to the lower back. In severe cases, these signs and symptoms can be peripheral, including **ecchymosis** (bruising), decrease in peripheral pulses, and embolic phenomenon in the toes. Aneurysms less than 4 cm in diameter are managed conservatively and hardly ever rupture, and those greater than 8 cm have a 50% chance of rupturing. Surgical intervention is dependent on the age of the patient, his or her general health, and the size of the aneurysm. Clinicians suspecting a **AAA** in a patient should refer them for further study because this condition may need urgent attention.

Preparation

Identify the following skeletal landmarks (N248; C267):

Xiphisternal joint
Costal margin
Anterior superior iliac spine
Pubic tubercle
Pubic symphysis
Arcuate line

Anatomic Overview

The basic vertebrate body plan has been described as *a tube within a tube.* On lateral folding of the embryo, the body wall encases a body cavity—the coelom—forming the outer tube. Suspended within is the gut tube coursing from head to tail. The gut tube is suspended from the dorsal body wall by a reflection of the mesothelium that lines the abdominal cavity, the dorsal mesentery. The smooth muscle of the gut tube derives from the visceral (splancnic) layer of the lateral plate mesoderm.

Ancillary organs, such as the liver and pancreas, form within the mesentery as outgrowths of the gastrointestinal (GI) track. Twisting of the mesentery and organs obscures the original bilateral symmetry of the organs, resulting in the liver lying to the right and the stomach and spleen lying to the left (Figure 8-1).

Dissection

Make a midline incision through the linea alba extending from sternum to pubis, making a slight detour circumventing the umbilicus.

Cut the abdominal muscles from the costal margin, and **reflect** them laterally.

Examine the abdominal organs in situ (N269; G2.18; GY142, 143; C204, 205). **Observe** the **greater omentum,** and **explore** the recesses of the **peritoneal cavity. Note** that some organs (e.g., stomach, jejunum, ileum, transverse colon, sigmoid colon)

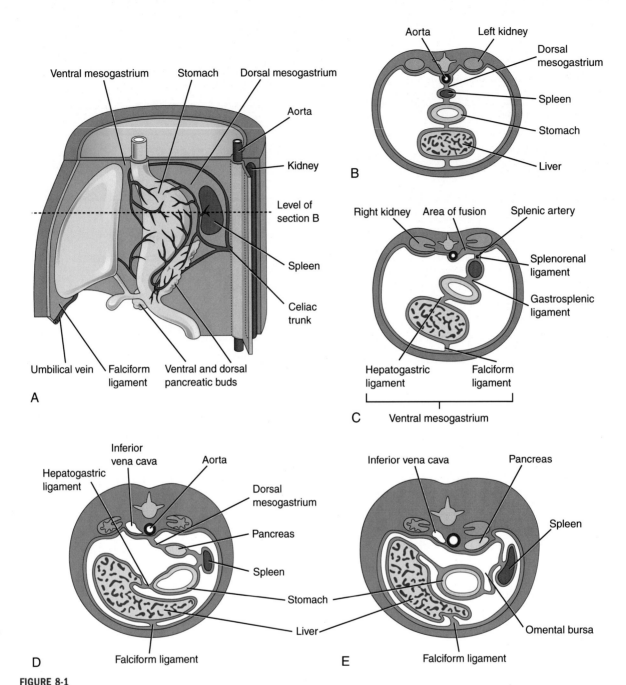

FIGURE 8-1

Embryonic rotation of the gut and ancillary organs of the abdomen, resulting in the adult positions of the organs. **A,** Lateral view of the left side of the liver, stomach, pancreas, and spleen. **B,** Transverse section at the level indicated in **A,** illustrating their relationships to the dorsal and ventral mesenteries. **C,** Transverse section of the fetus showing fusion of the dorsal mesogastrium to the posterior peritoneum. **D,** Movement of liver to the right and the stomach to the left. **E,** Observe the fusion of the mesogastrium to the posterior body wall, resulting in the pancreas becoming retroperitoneal. *(From Moore K, Persaud TVN: Before we are born: essentials of embryology and birth defects, ed 7, Philadelphia, 2008, WB Saunders.)*

are nearly completely encompassed by visceral peritoneum and may be suspended by a reflection of peritoneum called a **mesentery**. By contrast, some organs (e.g., kidneys, pancreas, duodenum, ascending and descending colon) appear to be adherent to the posterior body wall, with peritoneum only on their anterior surfaces. These organs are said to be **retroperitoneal.** Study their relationships in cross-section (**N342, 349; G2.21; GY176; C258-263**).

Tie off the esophagus inferior to the diaphragm.

Tie it off a second time 2 cm below the first, and **cut** the esophagus between the ligatures. **Repeat** this process at the rectum as far caudally as possible.

The goal is to remove the GI tract and ancillary organs as a single *pluck*. The organs that develop within the posterior body wall (e.g., kidneys, aorta, inferior vena cava) are termed **primarily retroperitoneal** and will be left in abdomen.

> **TIP** The ascending and descending colons are secondarily retroperitoneal (Figure 8-2). When separating the colon from the body wall, take care to avoid separating deep to the renal fascia and reflecting the kidneys unwittingly at this time.

Organs associated with the GI tract that are **secondarily retroperitoneal** will be removed. The peritoneum that holds them fixed to the posterior body wall will be cut, as will any structures that span between the body wall and the GI tract, such as **branches of the abdominal aorta** (N274; G2.62, 2.63; GY176; C240).

> **TIP** The venous drainage flows into the hepatic portal vein (N312; G 2.60; GY170) and then into the liver and therefore need not be cut. The inferior vena cava (IVC) is often encompassed by the liver. Therefore a short segment of the IVC may need to be excised with the liver to free it.

Begin at the rectum, and **pull** the GI tract upward, cutting the sigmoid mesocolon and the inferior mesenteric artery close to the aorta (N307; G2.44; GY160; C230, 232). **Free** the ascending and descending colons (N274; G2.62, 2.63; GY176; C240).

Cut the **root of the mesentery. Free** the duodenum.

Cut the superior mesenteric artery (N306; G2.39; GY154; C230). **Free** the pancreas and spleen (N292; G2.56; C210).

Cut the celiac trunk (N305; G2.29, 2.34; GY147, 150; C207). The liver may encompass the inferior vena cava. **Free** it and **cut** the hepatic veins (N287; G2.45, 2.46; GY162, 163; C217) and the **coronary and triangular ligaments** (Figure 8-3).

Examine the isolated GI tract, and **appreciate** the topographic relationships of the organs before placing it in a plastic bag.

Observe:

Liver, which lies in the upper right quadrant against the diaphragm. Note the bare area between the **coronary ligaments.** These ligaments are reinforced reflections of the peritoneum that suspend the heavy liver. The **hepatic portal vein** conveys blood from the intestines and spleen to the liver.

Gallbladder, which extends below the inferior border of the liver. The dark green stain is from bile. Check the gallbladder for stones.

Stomach

Intestines

Spleen

Pancreas

Aortic branches

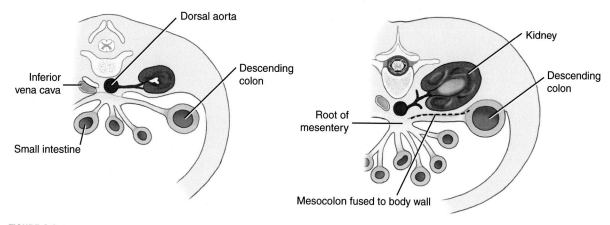

FIGURE 8-2

The kidneys develop within the posterior body wall and are therefore primarily retroperitoneal. The descending colon becomes attached to the posterior body wall and is therefore secondarily retroperitoneal.

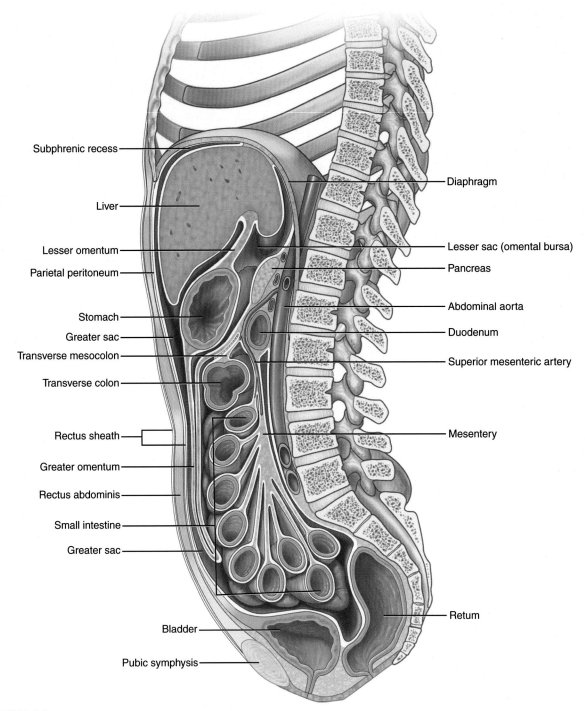

Subphrenic recess

Liver

Lesser omentum

Parietal peritoneum

Stomach

Greater sac

Transverse mesocolon

Transverse colon

Rectus sheath

Greater omentum

Rectus abdominis

Small intestine

Greater sac

Bladder

Pubic symphysis

Diaphragm

Lesser sac (omental bursa)

Pancreas

Abdominal aorta

Duodenum

Superior mesenteric artery

Mesentery

Retum

FIGURE 8-3

Midsagittal section through the abdomen. *(From Drake R et al:* Gray's atlas of anatomy, *Philadelphia, 2008, Churchill Livingstone.)*

Exercises

1. Label on the figure below the branches of the abdominal aorta.

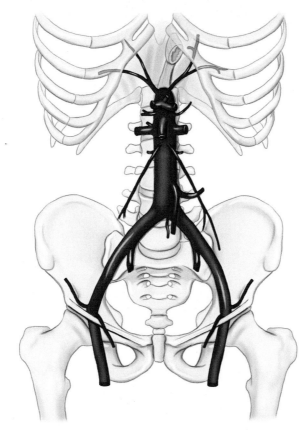

2. Label on the figure below the cross-section through the upper abdomen.

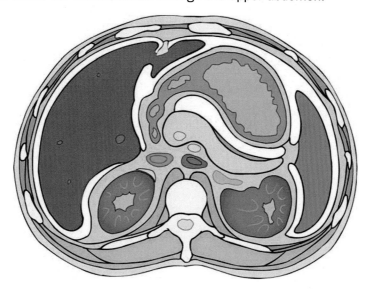

3. A perforated gastric ulcer of the posterior stomach wall ejects digestive juices into the lesser omental bursa. What retroperitoneal organs are at risk from the corrosive stomach fluids?

4. Label on the figure below the tributaries of the hepatic portal vein.

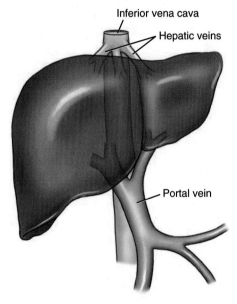

Inferior vena cava

Hepatic veins

Portal vein

LAB EXPLORATION **9**

Diaphragm, Kidneys, and Bladder

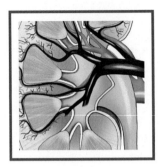

LAB OBJECTIVES

In this lab the muscular boundary between the abdomen and thorax will be examined and the anatomy and topographic relationships of the kidney defined. On completion of this lab the student will be able to:

- Describe the development, attachments, and innervation of the abdominal diaphragm.
- Define the fascial coverings of the kidney.
- Identify the anatomy of the kidney, course of the ureters, and position of the bladder relative to the peritoneum.

CASE STUDY

Difficulty Breathing

Andy is a 17 **y/o** patient who was involved in an **MVA** while riding his motorcycle. His front wheel slipped on gravel while he was negotiating a turn, and he struck a utility pole. He was rushed to the **ER**, where a computerized tomographic **(CT)** study indicated a complete transection of the spinal cord secondary to a displaced fracture of thoracic vertebrae five **(T5)** that left him paralyzed below that level. He was admitted for surgery, where he was stabilized and fused at levels T4 through T6 and fitted for a thoracolumbosacral orthosis to help in the healing process. He was temporarily placed on a ventilator because his tidal volume **(V$_t$)** was marginal. He was successfully weaned from the ventilator 5 days later and was moved to the rehabilitation floor for aggressive intervention.

Identification of the Anatomy

The crucial portion of this dissection is to identify the phrenic and vagus nerves and to trace them from their origin to the effector organs. These nerves are

paramount in the function of the diaphragm and heart. (Review Lab Exploration 6.)

Appreciate the following structures during dissection:

Costal margins
Left and right diaphragmatic crura
Central tendon
Origin and insertion of the diaphragm proper
Esophagus
Aorta
Inferior vena cava
Lumbar vertebrae and sacral promontory

Questions

1. Given the level of the injury, what muscles, sensations, and bodily functions are lost in this patient?
2. Dependent on the level of the injury, the patient with spinal cord injury **(SCI)** will have difficulty breathing. Can you postulate why an SCI will be a problem for this patient?

79

3. Describe the action of the diaphragm during the ventilation process. How can a clinician assist this patient in improving his ventilation dynamics?

Discussion

Many SCIs involve adolescents who use poor judgment involving speed, alcohol, and drugs. Some SCIs do not result in complete transection the spinal cord, and the patient has some function left, dependent on the level. In this case the patient's transection is *complete,* and he has lost all function below T4. Given that the ventilation action of the diaphragm is controlled by the phrenic nerve (C3-C5), the lungs still functions, but the patient will not benefit from the intercostal action to enhance the *pump-handle* and *bucket-handle* mechanisms discussed earlier. The chest wall rise will be limited, and the patient will need to use the accessory musculature of the upper trunk and neck to assist in inhalation. Numerous techniques in the clinician's armamentarium can be used to enhance muscle action of the diaphragm, including muscular training and abdominal compression binders; even inspiratory weights to assist in diaphragmatic strengthening have been used. The patient with an SCI special case must be monitored closely in the hospital setting to ensure progressive gains and the best recovery possible.

Preparation

Identify the following skeletal landmarks (N248; C267):

> **Xiphisternal joint**
> **Costal margin**
> **Transverse processes of lumbar vertebrae**
> **Sacral promontory**
> **Iliac crest**
> **Anterior superior iliac spine**
> **Pectineal line**
> **Arcuate line**
> **Ala (wing) of ilium**

Anatomic Overview

The diaphragm begins as a mass of mesoderm cranial to the pericardium. The head fold develops during the fourth week, which swings the mass of mesoderm inferior to the heart and is called the **septum transversum** (Figure 9-1). This structure is destined to become the central tendon of the diaphragm. As the mass of mesoderm passes beneath the cervical region, it receives myoblasts from the C3 through C5

hypomeres. Thus the myoblasts receive their innervation from ventral rami of cervical spinal nerves C3 through C5, forming the **phrenic nerve.** The myoblasts and their nerves reach the septum transversum via the **pleuropericardial membranes.** Hence the adult phrenic nerve lies within the fibrous pericardium between the mediastinal pleura and the serous pericardium. Continued growth causes the diaphragm to descend until the dorsal portion reaches the level of the first lumbar vertebra.

Additional components of the diaphragm are contributed by the **pleuroperitoneal membranes** (these membranes represent a relatively small portion of the adult diaphragm), the **mesentery of the esophagus,** and the **body wall** (Figure 9-2). The inner portion of the body wall splits away and contributes to the periphery of the diaphragm, forming the **costodiaphragmatic recess.** This portion of the diaphragm receives its sensory innervation from branches of the lower six or seven intercostal nerves.

The kidneys begin their development within the **intermediate mesoderm** in the posterior body wall as the third in a series of successive nephric structures of increasingly advanced design—the pronephros, mesonephros, and metanephros. The **ureteric bud** induces differentiation of the **metanephric blastema,** and vice versa, in the region of the sacrum. The ureteric bud repeatedly bifurcates to form the **renal pelvis, calyces,** and **collecting ducts.** Simultaneously, the metanephric blastema gives rise to the nephron-containing **cortex** of the kidney. (Figure 9-3). The kidneys then ascend to the lumbar region and are repeatedly revascularized by a series of aortic sprouts along the way. If one of these transient renal arteries fails to regress, an accessory renal artery may be present (N333). Should a kidney fail to ascend, it may remain adjacent to the sacrum as a pelvic kidney. Rarely, the inferior poles of the metanephroi may fuse, forming a *horseshoe kidney* (G2.69; C234).

Dissection

Now turn your attention to the **thoracic diaphragm** (N195; G2.74; GY175; C252). Identify the following:

> **Central tendon**
> **Cava canal**
> **Esophageal hiatus**
> **Right and left crura**
> **Median, medial and lateral arcuate ligaments**
> **Phrenic nerves**

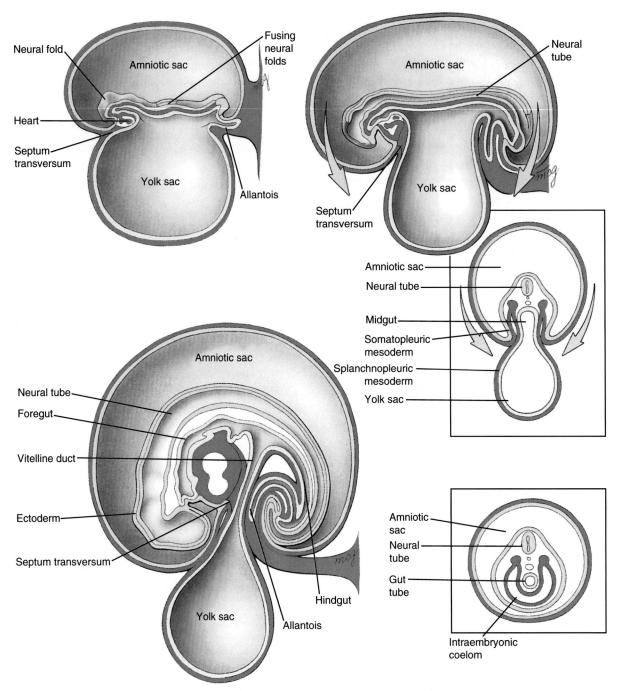

FIGURE 9-1
Migration of the septum transversum during cranial folding. *(From Larsen W: Human embryology, ed 3, Philadelphia, 2001, Churchill Livingstone.)*

Examine the posterior abdominal body wall. **Identify** the remains of the parietal peritoneum after removal of the GI tract (**N329; G2.62; C243**). Deep to the peritoneum, over the posterior body wall, is the **retroperitoneal space** containing the **pararenal fat** (**N342; G2.64, 2.71; GY176; C259**). It extends lateral and posterior to the kidney.

Scrape through the layer of fat to reach the **perirenal (Gerota's) fascia**. The perirenal fascia encompasses a layer of **perirenal fat** that surrounds the kidney and **suprarenal gland.**

Free the right kidney from its renal fascia, and **examine** it in situ, identifying its blood supply (**N332, 341; G2.63; GY180, 183; C243**).

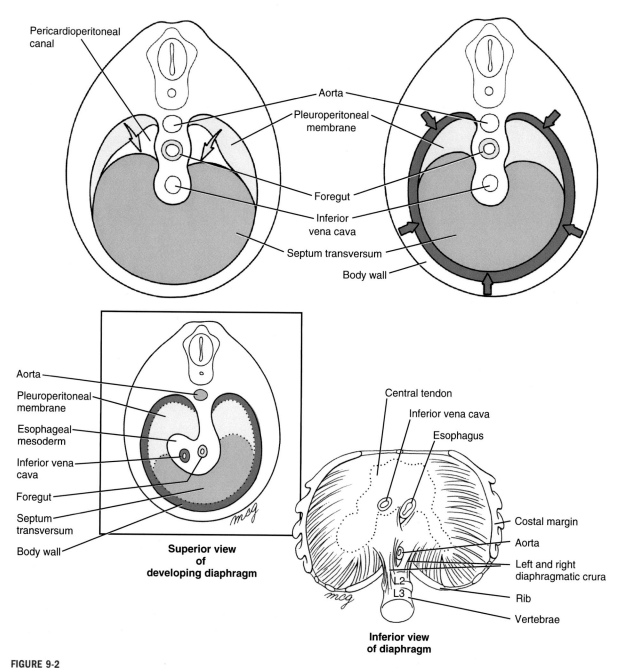

FIGURE 9-2

Contributions to the formation of the diaphragm. *(From Larsen W:* Human embryology, *ed 3, Philadelphia, 2001, Churchill Livingstone.)*

Use a sectioning knife rather than a scalpel to **divide** it evenly along a coronal plane, leaving the ureter and renal vessels intact and attached.

Examine the gross structure of the kidney (**N334, 335; G2.66; GY178; C245, 247**) (Figure 9-4). Notice the fibrous **renal capsule** of dense, irregular connective tissue. **Identify** the outer **cortex** and **renal columns,** the tightly packed collecting tubules forming the **medullary pyramids,** and the **papillae** projecting into the **calyces.** The calyces coalesce into the renal pelvis, which, in turn, tapers into the ureter.

Trace the ureter across the **psoas muscle** to the **urinary bladder,** which lies below the **peritoneum** (**N274; G2.63; GY183; C243**). **Incise** the superior surface of the bladder, and **examine** its interior. Note the thickness of the smooth muscle wall of the bladder.

Locate the smooth **trigone** defined by the two orifices of the ureters and the **urethra. Insert** a probe into a ureter, and note the angle it passes through the wall of the bladder (**N366; G3.24; GY218; C304**).

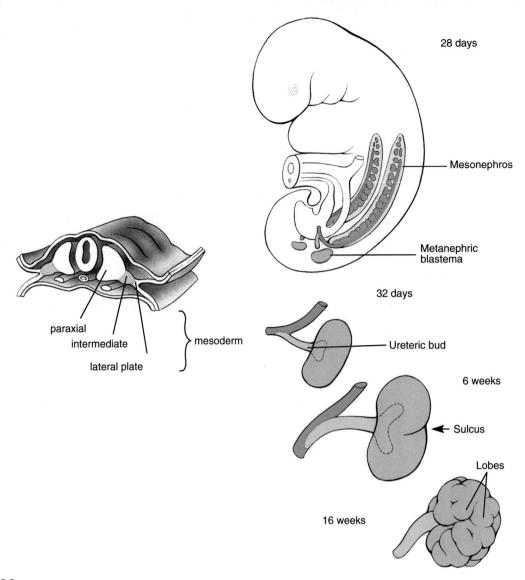

28 days

Mesonephros

Metanephric
blastema

paraxial
intermediate
lateral plate
mesoderm

32 days

Ureteric bud

6 weeks

Sulcus

Lobes

16 weeks

FIGURE 9-3

The urogenital system derives from the intermediate mesoderm. The adult kidney develops from the metanephric blastema. *(From Larsen W:* Human embryology, *3e, Philadelphia, 2001, Churchill Livingstone.)*

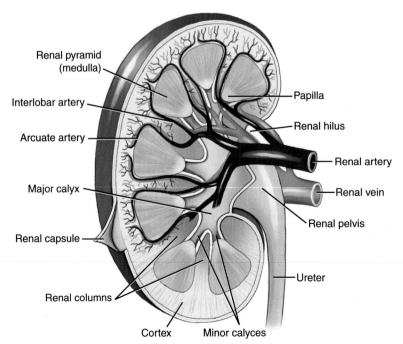

Renal pyramid
(medulla)

Interlobar artery

Arcuate artery

Major calyx

Renal capsule

Renal columns

Cortex

Minor calyces

Papilla

Renal hilus

Renal artery

Renal vein

Renal pelvis

Ureter

FIGURE 9-4

Coronal section through the kidney.

Exercises

1. In this inferior view of the costal margin, sketch in and label the key features of the abdominal diaphragm, including the central tendons, hiatuses, crura, and ligaments.

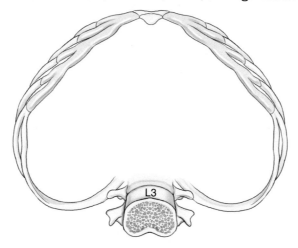

2. On the outline of a computed tomographic (CT) scan of the upper abdomen, identify and label the depicted structures.

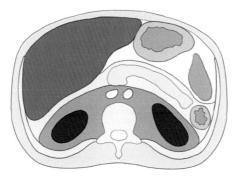

3. Why might neck pain be symptomatic of irritation of the diaphragm?

4. Why might spasm in the diaphragm cause a "side-ache" or runner's stitch, i.e. pain in the lower thoracic bodywall?

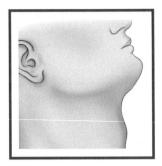

Triangles of the Neck

> **LAB OBJECTIVES**
>
> In this lab we will explore the superficial boundaries of the triangles of the neck and their contents. On completion the student should be able to:
>
> * Define the boundaries and contents of the triangles of the anterior neck.
> * Describe the attachments, innervations, and actions of the muscles of the visceral neck.
> * Describe the organization and distribution of the cervical plexus.
> * Define dermatomes and correlate and contrast them with named cutaneous nerve fields.
> * Distinguish the fundamental structural differences between large arteries and veins.

CASE STUDY

The Stinger

Kayla, a 23 **y/o** pole vault competitor at the collegiate level, visits the **OP** bumps and bruises clinic for athletes on Saturday morning after a Friday night track meet. Her **CC** relates to weakness and some numbness and tingling **(NT)** of her entire right upper extremity. Her subjective information indicates that she missed the pit on a vault and came down near the hard edge of the track, with the primary impact on the top of her **R** shoulder and the same side of the neck. She states that she felt the entire arm "go to sleep" and was unable to move it. Kayla suggested that the sensation lasted approximately 20 minutes, and then some feeling and strength returned. Her examination today revealed minor bruising on the **R** acromion process, with minimal edema on the same side trapezius. Grip strength was decreased on the **R** compared with the **L,** and she was unable to raise the **R** arm actively above her head, but her elbow, wrist, and hand **AROM** were normal.

Identification of the Anatomy

The cervical plexus becomes important because it is sometimes implicated in stretch injuries or compression syndromes resulting from muscle tightness and spasticity, as well as lesions to the C1-C4 vertebra. The dissection should allow for specific isolation of the muscles and nerve roots of this region.

Appreciate the following structure during dissection:

> Clavicle, first rib, and sternum
> Sternocleidomastoid
> Scalene grouping
> Upper portion of the brachial plexus
> Subclavian artery and vein

Questions

1. If the head abruptly moves away from the shoulder or the shoulder is depressed beyond the normal limit, what structures may be temporarily compromised?

2. Given Kayla's signs and symptoms, what structures were clearly altered as a result of the fall?
3. Can you explain why her feeling returned relatively quickly and why the strength in her arm took longer to return?

Discussion

The cause of this injury is a depressed shoulder with the head in the opposite direction, which places an unusual load on the cervical and brachial plexi tension. In sports medicine language, this condition is commonly known as a *stinger* and can render an athlete incapable of completing a game or an event. The term *neuropraxia* is sometimes used to suggest that the nerve *sheath* is slightly stretched and not ruptured. This stretching of the cervical or brachial plexi (see Exploration Lab 11) immediately and temporarily shuts down both motor and sensory function. In addition, a transient ischemic response to these nerves occurs, which slows blood flow, adding to the problem. Most stingers respond well to rest and protective measures during play. However, transient muscle weakness and **NT** may linger for days or longer. In more severe cases, the nerve roots, trunks, or cords may actually rupture, which leads to serious injury and possible paralysis of certain arm and shoulder functions. The mechanism of injury in Kayla's case is very similar to that seen in football players when they execute a tackle or a block using poor mechanics. The same injury may also be the result of wearing shoulder pads that do not fit properly. The only difference is that Kayla used her body weight to initiate the tension rather than another player.

Preparation

Identify the bony landmarks of the anterior neck (N13; G8.4; GY489):

> **Mastoid process (temporal bone)**
> **Styloid process (temporal bone)**
> **Mandible**
> **Digastric fossa**
> **Hyoid bone**
> **Clavicle**
> **Sternum**

Anatomic Overview

In this exploration, we encounter another aspect of the distribution of **ventral rami of spinal nerves.** In the cervical region, as also in the lumbosacral region, the ventral rami form a **plexus** (L. *braid*), in which fibers are exchanged between ventral rami.

The **cervical plexus** is formed by the first four cervical ventral rami. The brachial plexus is formed by the last four cervical and first thoracic ventral rami.

We have learned that a **dermatome** is defined as that area of skin innervated by a single spinal nerve. However, in the region of a plexus, the exchange of nerve fibers between levels results in named cutaneous nerve branches that contain axons originating from multiple spinal levels. These **cutaneous nerves** serve a restricted region of several adjacent dermatomes. Sensory deficits that follow this pattern are indicative of *peripheral* nerve lesions.

In the neck, we encounter further examples of major arteries and veins, such as the **common carotid artery** and the **internal jugular vein.** These vessels differ noticeably in texture and appearance, which will assist you in their identification (Figure 10-1, *A*). These differences are basically responses to differences in pressure encountered by the respective vessels. Arteries are relatively thick walled, with variable quantities of elastic fibers. The principal difference lies in the intermediate layer, the **tunica media,** which contains smooth muscle, collagen, and elastin. Veins generally have larger diameter lumen than accompanying arteries. They have relatively thin walls with more collagen but less elastin and smooth muscle. Medium-size veins have **valves,** formed by pairs of semilunar extensions of the **tunica intima.** They prevent back flow of blood and build-up of pressure in distal veins, especially in the lower extremities. In the periphery, arteries travel together with veins and nerves, forming **neurovascular bundles** (Figure 10-1, *B*).

Dissection

Make a midline incision on the anterior neck from the **mentum** (chin) to the suprasternal notch.
Reflect and **remove** the skin flaps, taking care to leave the very superficial **playsma** in place (**N26; G8.1; GY492; C472**).
Clean its surface, and **note** the **supraclavicular nerves** emerging from below the inferior margin of the muscle (**N31; G8.1; GY494; C476**). These nerves are cutaneous nerves from the ventral rami of cervical spinal nerves (C3-C4), supplying sensation to the skin of the neck just above the clavicles (**N32; GY496**).
Reflect the platysma upward, tracing the supraclavicular nerves to the point where they emerge from under the posterior edge of the **sternocleidomastoid muscle.**

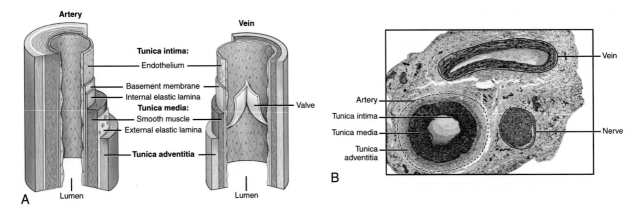

FIGURE 10-1

A, Sectioned artery and vein. **B,** Neurovascular bundle containing artery, vein, and nerve. *(Part B from Telser A et al: Elsevier's integrated histology, Philadelphia, 2007, Mosby.)*

The **posterior triangle** of the neck is bounded by the **trapezius,** the sternocleidomastoid and the clavicle **(G8.1; GY488; C471)** (Figure 10-2). It is further subdivided by the posterior belly of the **omohyoid** muscle into an occipital and a supraclavicular triangle. The posterior triangle is covered by an **investing fascia,** which is continuous with the epimysium, or deep fascia, of the trapezius and sternocleidomastoid muscles.

Use the scissor technique to isolate the nerves within this triangle:

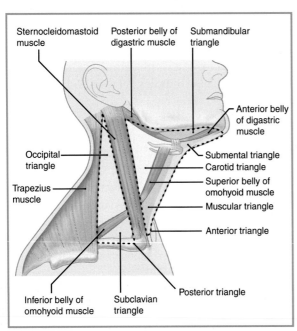

FIGURE 10-2

Major and minor triangles of the neck. *(From Moses KP et al: Atlas of clinical gross anatomy, Philadelphia, 2005, Mosby.)*

Accessory nerve (cranial nerve [CN] XI, C2, 3, 4). It runs on the **levator scapula muscle,** emerging from beneath the posterior border of the sternocleidomastoid and disappearing beneath the anterior border of the trapezius. It supplies motor innervation to the sternocleidomastoid and the trapezius.

Three additional cutaneous nerves radiate from the posterior border of the sternocleidomastoid in proximity to the CN XI. These branches arise from a loop between C2 and C3 ventral rami. This structure is part of the cervical plexus (Figure 10-3).

Lesser occipital nerve (C2-C3). It courses along or near the posterior border of the sternocleidomastoid to innervate the region of the scalp behind the ear.

Great auricular nerve (C2-C3). It ascends on the surface of the sternocleidomastoid alongside the external jugular vein.

Transverse cervical nerve (C2-C3). It courses transversely across the middle of the sternocleidomastoid to innervate the skin over the anterior triangle of the neck.

Remove the remaining investing fascia to expose the muscular floor of the posterior triangle.

Beginning at the apex of the triangle, **identify** the **splenius capitis, levator scapula, scalenus posterior, scalenus medius,** and **scalenus anterior** (N27; G8.5; GY492; C473). The attachments of these muscles will be examined more closely along with the remaining prevertebral muscles during a later exploration. Note the interval between the scalenus medius and scalenus anterior. Together with the first rib, they form the **interscalene triangle,** through which the **subclavian artery** and **brachial plexus** pass.

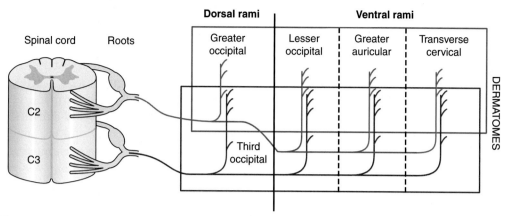

FIGURE 10-3

A portion of the cervical plexus illustrates the course and components of branches of the dorsal and ventral rami.

Should the triangle become narrowed as a result of anomalous muscle slips or cervical ribs, the artery or nerve may become compressed leading to ischemia or nerve dysfunction in the upper extremity.

Pull the sternocleidomastoid forward, and **note** the **phrenic nerve** (C3-C5) descending across the scalenus anterior and on into the thorax to innervate the diaphragm (**N32; G8.5; GY495**).

The **anterior triangle** of the neck is bounded by the sternocleidomastoid, the body of the mandible, and the anterior midline of the neck. The anterior triangle is further subdivided into the muscular, carotid, submandibular, and submental triangles. Note such visceral structures as the submandibular gland, thyroid cartilage, thyroid gland, common carotid artery, and internal jugular vein.

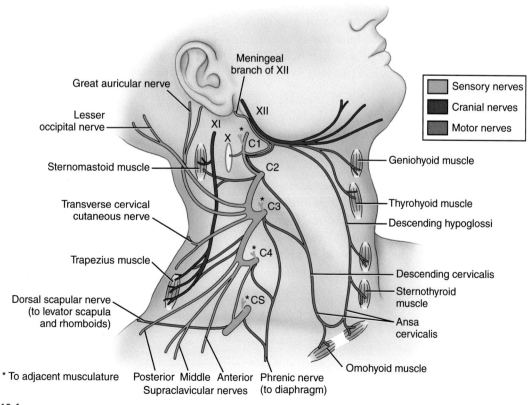

FIGURE 10-4

The cervical plexus.

Here, we focus our attention on the neuromuscular components of the anterior triangle.

Section the sternocleidomastoid muscle 1 to 2 cm above its attachment to the clavicle and sternum, and carefully **reflect** it laterally.

Use the scissor technique to find where the **accessory nerve** enters the deep surface of the muscle. The muscular triangle is separated from the carotid triangle by the **omohyoid** muscle. The remaining infrahyoid muscles include the **sternohyoid,** the **sternothyroid,** and the **thyrohyoid** muscles. These muscles receive motor innervation by ventral rami of cervical spinal nerves (C1-C3) via the **ansa cervicalis** (a portion of the cervical plexus).

To locate the ansa cervicalis, first palpate the **greater horns of the hyoid bone** between thumb and index finger. The **hypoglossal nerve** (CN XII) can be found immediately superior to it, passing deep to the **posterior belly of the digastric (N32; G8.10; GY494; C479, 480)** (Figure 10-4). Here the C1-C2 fibers leave as the **nerve to the thyrohyoid.**

Follow this nerve to the lateral border of the muscle.

Trace the hypoglossal nerve back to the superior root of the ansa cervicalis, the **decendens hypoglossi** (C1). The superior root joins the inferior root, the **decendens cervicalis** (C2-C3), to form the ansa (L. *loop, handle*). **Trace** the nerve branches from the ansa cervicalis to the infrahyoid muscles.

Four muscles, called the suprahyoid muscles **(N29; G8.10; GY493; C482, 483)**, are located above the hyoid bone and serve to anchor it to the skull. These muscles are actually muscles of the head and thus receive innervation from cranial nerves. The first muscle is the **digastric muscle.** As its name implies, it has two bellies joined by an intermediate tendon attached to the hyoid bone. The two bellies receive distinct innervations. The anterior belly is innervated by the **mylohyoid nerve,** a branch of the inferior alveolar nerve (in turn,

a branch of the trigeminal nerve, CN V). The posterior belly is innervated by the facial nerve (CN VII). The **stylohyoid** is a narrow slip of a muscle lying parallel to the posterior belly of the digastric, also innervated by the facial nerve. The belly is perforated by the intermediate tendon of the digastric. The **mylohyoid** muscles form the floor of the buccal cavity and are innervated by the mylohyoid nerve. They are united at the midline by a median fibrous **raphe.**

Divide the raphe with a scalpel to expose the fourth suprahyoid muscle, the **geniohyoid.** This muscle is the apparent exception in that it is innervated by a branch of C1 that travels on the hypoglossal nerve.

Review the attachments, innervation, and actions of these muscles.

Clinical Note

Wry neck

The sternocleidomastoid muscle is a prominent landmark in the anterior neck. If the muscle shortens, either through formation of a fibrotic tumor or by spasm, the face is drawn upward and away from the effected side. This condition is called **torticollis,** or wry neck. A potential complication of vaginal delivery, *muscular torticollis,* occurs when excessive traction is placed on the infant's neck. A resulting hematoma in the torn muscle is invaded by fibrous connective tissue, shortening the muscle. Abnormal tonicity, known as *spasmodic torticollis,* results from repeated chronic contraction of the sternocleidomastoid and trapezius. It is usually psychogenic in origin. Sectioning of the spinal part of the spinal accessory nerve may be necessitated. In some cases, Botox® injections (botulism toxin) may be administered to decrease the spasms. *What postural changes would result from the denervation of muscles supplied by the spinal accessory?*

Exercises

1. Draw in and label the boundaries of the triangles of the neck.

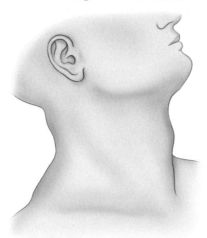

2. Draw in the dermatomes of the anterior neck and upper thorax.

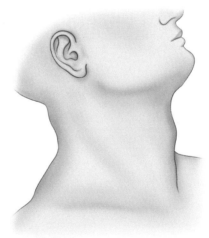

3. Draw in the cutaneous nerve fields.

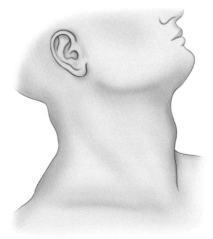

4. Label on the figure below the major structures of the visceral neck as seen in cross-section.

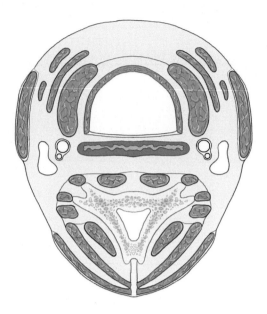

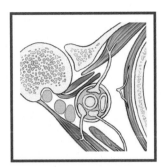

Pectoral Region and Axilla

LAB OBJECTIVES

In this lab the anatomy of the pectoral region and contents of the axilla (armpit) will be considered. This region is the nexus of the upper extremity and torso, transmitting neurovascular structures from the neck and thorax into the upper extremity. On completion of this exercise the student should be able to:

- Identify the bony landmarks and ligaments of the scapula, clavicle and sternum, and proximal humerus.
- Identify the extrinsic limb muscles attached to the anterior chest wall.
- Define the boundaries and contents of the axilla.
- Identify the branches of the subclavian and axillary arteries.
- Identify the roots, trunks, divisions, cords, and branches of the brachial plexus.

CASE STUDY

Dangerous Fall

Ursula is an 82 **y/o** resident in a long-term care **(LTC)** facility affiliated with a hospital. She is independent with self-care activities and is not suffering from dementia. She briefly lost her balance on the way back to her room from dinner and fell *lightly* against the wall outside her room but did not fall completely to the ground; thus she proceeded back to bed. At bedside, she notified the nurse on duty with her call button. On examination, Ursula **c/o** severe pain of the **L** shoulder and noted that she was unable to raise her left arm. In sitting position, Ursula guards her shoulder by supporting it with the other hand. The patient exhibits a noticeable deformity of the **L** clavicle, and the corresponding shoulder is lower than the **R.** The area is tender to palpation and discolored, and she **c/o** shortness of breath **(SOB)**. The attending physician is called, and she is taken to the hospital for radiographic examination and evaluation.

Identification of the Anatomy

The shoulder girdle dissection is complex because of the constellation of nerves, muscles, bony prominences, and vessels housed in and around several joint articulations. When dissecting through the muscular tissues and fascia, be careful to proceed slowly because nerves and vessels lie in close proximity to deeper structures. The shoulder girdle is composed of three true joints (acromioclavicular, glenohumeral, and sternoclavicular) and one pseudo joint (scapulothoracic), and these joints allow for movements that create proximal stability for distal precision movements of the forearm and hand. Also note the proximal to distal course of the nerves of the brachial plexus. At times, identifying the nerves from distal branches to proximal divisions, cords, and trunks may be easier.

Appreciate the following structures during dissection:

Clavicle
First and second ribs
Acromion and coracoid processes
Sternoclavicular junction
Pectoralis major and minor
Subclavius muscle
Brachial plexus
Thoracic outlet and contents
Rotator cuff musculature

Questions

1. In the geriatric population, falling is a constant fear. Can you describe some of the other factors that predispose older adults to falls?
2. The patient's **Dx** was a fractured clavicle and rib two and three. Given that the patient did not fall to the floor, what other issues may have predisposed this patient to fracture?
3. Clavicle healing is difficult, and issues with malunion and with cosmetic deformity are almost always present. Why is this the case?

Discussion

The ambulatory elderly person in extended-care facilities is at great risk for falling because of a constellation of factors. Poor eyesight, weak muscles, joint deformities, vestibular issues, and the effect of poly pharmacy are only a few. In addition, the elderly women are prone to osteoporosis, which complicates matters when they do fall. The unfortunate sequelae of this patient is all too common, given that fractures in the elderly persons, especially fractures in the lower extremity, decrease their mobility, which, in turn, invites opportunistic infections to take hold, eventually leading to pneumonia and death. This patient also had a closed **pneumothorax** secondary to the third-rib puncturing her apical segment of the **L** lung. Fall-prevention programs are essential for geriatric persons, and the rehabilitation professional should be actively engaged in promoting them.

Preparation

On the articulated skeleton, note the relationship of the elements of the pectoral girdle to the rib cage (N185; G1.9; GY57; C104). The skeletal boundaries of the **axilla** include the **subscapular fossa**, the **clavicle**, the **ribs**, and the **intertubercular sulcus** (bicipital groove) of the **humerus** (N420; G6.1, 6.31; GY351-335; C76, 77). *What is the relationship of the axilla to the superior thoracic aperture and the cervical region?*

Identify on the **scapula** (N420, 421; G6.1, 6.31; GY353; C76):

Acromion process
Coracoid process
Subscapular fossa

Identify on the **clavicle** (N419; GY354; C104):

Acromial end
Sternal end
Trapezoid line
Conoid tubercle
Impression for costoclavicular ligament

Identify on the **sternum** (N419; GY354; C105):

Manubrium
Jugular notch
Sternal angle (angle of Louie)

Anatomic Overview

The developing upper limb bud forms as an outgrowth of the body wall. Much of its connective tissue—bone, fascia, and vessels—arise from the somatic layer of the lateral plate mesoderm. However, the muscles derive from the hypomeres of dermatomes C5-T1 and therefore are accompanied by branches of the ventral rami of these spinal nerves. As the cells of the hypomeres enter the limb bud, they segregate dorsally and ventrally into extensors and flexors (Figure 11-1). Their accompanying nerves are called dorsal and ventral division nerves, respectively.

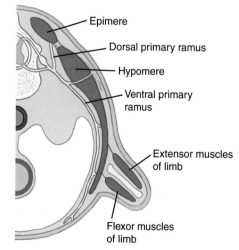

FIGURE 11-1

Transverse section of the embryonic limb bud. Note the segregation of myoblasts from the hypomere into dorsal and ventral divisions correlated with the extensor and flexor compartments respectively.

The fact of this division and compartmentalization of the muscles of the limb can be used to advantage by simplifying the learning of the innervation of the muscles of the limbs. Rather than memorizing individual muscle innervations, particular nerves are associated with entire or even multiple compartments, innervating all the muscles located within those compartments. Figure 11-2 provides an overview of the pattern of innervation of the upper extremity.

Dissection

Place the cadaver in a supine position. Before removing the remaining skin from the arm, **trace** the superficial veins, and **review** the cutaneous nerves (**N479, 481; G6.6; G6.10; GY381, 384; C27, 30, 31**).

Identify the **cephalic vein** within the **deltopectoral groove.** Isolate and leave it in place. **Note** that the **basilic vein** passes under the deep fascia of the arm approximately midway between the axilla and the elbow; also note the pattern of distribution of the cutaneous nerves on the anterior aspect of the arm and their respective fields of sensory innervation. **Delineate** the area of skin supplied by the **medial cutaneous nerve** of the forearm which emerges from beneath the deep fascia alongside the basilic vein.

Review the attachments of the **pectoralis major.** It forms the anterior wall of the axilla.

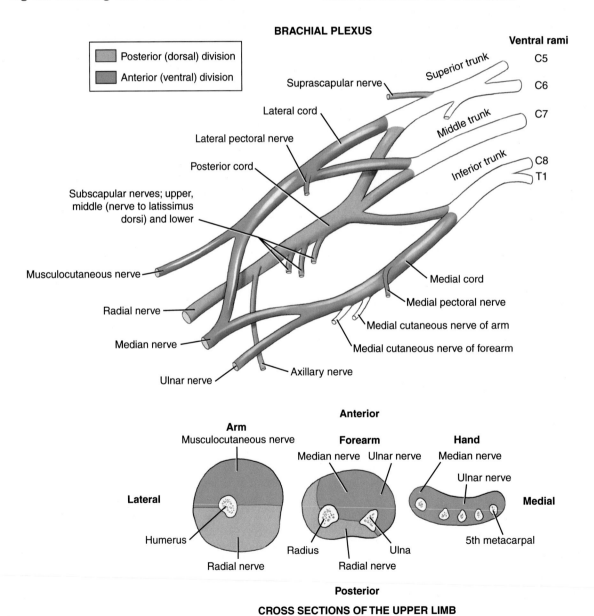

FIGURE 11-2
Organization and distribution of the brachial plexus.

Define the **deltopectoral triangle** and its content. The base of the triangle is at the clavicle, and its sides are bounded by the pectoralis major and deltoid muscles.

Cut the pectoralis major approximately 1 cm from its sternocostal and clavicular attachments, and **reflect** it laterally if not already done.

Identify the **medial pectoral** (C8-T1) and **lateral pectoral** (C5-T7) nerves (N188; G6.24; GY361; C15).

TIP The medial and lateral pectoral nerves are named for the cords of the brachial plexus from which they arise. They switch relative positions as they approach the pectoral muscles.

Observe that the **clavipectoral fascia** is continuous with the epimysium of the **pectoralis minor** and the **subclavius muscles** (N428; G6.11, 6.18; GY631; C15).

Cut the pectoralis minor 1 cm from its costal attachment, and **reflect** it laterally.

Clean away the remains of the clavipectoral fascia.

The **axilla** is a pyramidal space, the base of which is formed by the skin of the armpit (N429; G6.19-21; GY361; C18). Note the continuity of the posterior triangle of the neck with the axilla. *What neurovascular structures found in the posterior triangle of the neck continue into the axilla?* Three muscular structures are found within the axilla: the **long head of the biceps brachii tendon** (within the intertubercular sulcus), the **short head of the biceps brachii tendon,** and the **coracobrachialis** (Figure 11-3).

The remaining visceral contents of the axilla are surrounded by a sheath of connective tissue. These structures are the **axillary artery** and **vein** and the cords of the **brachial plexus.** Note that the contents of the **axillary sheath** pass over the first rib and under the clavicle.

Resect the middle third of the clavicle. The **axillary vein** consists of a complex network of channels that will have to be removed.

Clean away the axillary sheath, and define the branches of the **subclavian** and **axillary arteries** (N427; G6.21; GY368; C17):

Thyrocervical trunk
Suprascapular, transverse cervical, and **inferior thyroid**
Dorsal scapular (usually a branch of the transverse cervical)
Thoracoacromial:
  Pectoral
  Deltoid
  Acromial
  Clavicular
Lateral thoracic
Subscapular—thoracodorsal
Circumflex scapular
Medial and lateral humeral circumflex

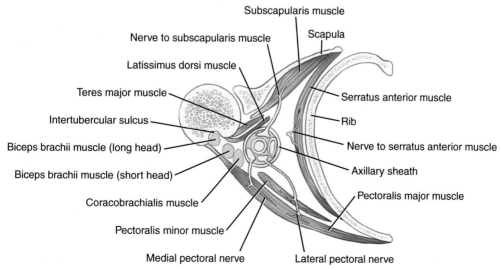

Subscapularis muscle
Nerve to subscapularis muscle
Scapula
Latissimus dorsi muscle
Teres major muscle
Serratus anterior muscle
Intertubercular sulcus
Rib
Biceps brachii muscle (long head)
Nerve to serratus anterior muscle
Biceps brachii muscle (short head)
Axillary sheath
Coracobrachialis muscle
Pectoralis major muscle
Pectoralis minor muscle
Medial pectoral nerve
Lateral pectoral nerve

FIGURE 11-3
Transverse section through the axilla.

Cervical rib syndrome—thoracic outlet syndrome

Cervical rib syndrome is the most common neurovascular compression at the neck base. It occurs in approximately 0.5% of people: bilateral in one half, unilateral in one half, slightly more common on the right side than the left side, and more common in women than in men. Occasionally, an additional rib is present on the seventh cervical vertebra. The rib narrows the interval between scalenes and creates a higher barrier over which nerves and vessels must pass (N173). Compression is worsened by shoulder sag (e.g., in elderly or muscle weakness) or carrying heavy object in hand or on shoulders (heavy luggage in airport, child on shoulders to watch a parade). Levels C8 to T1 are most commonly affected, resulting in pain and paresthesia along the ulnar nerve course. Patient may experience weakness, numbness, cold sensation, and clumsiness in the hand. The condition is indicated by palpable cervical rib, tender brachial plexus distribution, muscle weakness and atrophy, especially the interosseus muscles and hypothenar muscles. Circulatory insufficiency may also be present, including swelling, cold sensation, and distal cyanosis. Such vascular compromise is a form of *impingement syndrome*.

BRACHIAL PLEXUS

(N429, 430; G6.22; GY369; C18)

Clean the nerves of the brachial plexus, and trace them proximally to the **interscalene triangle.** The complex nomenclature of the brachial plexus can be a bit daunting. Think of this structure as an inverted tree, beginning with roots that coalesce into trunks, then divide into divisions, then unite into cords, and finally divide into terminal branches *(unite, divide, unite, divide).*

Roots

Identify the roots as the five ventral rami of C5 through T1 *(not to be confused with the dorsal and ventral roots of the spinal nerves!).* Here are found the **dorsal scapular nerve** (C5) to the rhomboids and the **long thoracic nerve** (C5-C7) to the serratus anterior.

Trunks

The ventral rami of C5-C6 unite to form the **superior trunk,** which gives off the **suprascapular nerve** (C5-C6) to the supraspinatus and infraspinatus

muscles and the **nerve to the subclavius** (C5-C6). The ventral ramus of C7 remains single as the **middle trunk.** The ventral rami of C8 and T1 unite to form the **inferior trunk.**

Divisions

Next, the trunks segregate into **anterior** and **posterior divisions** associated with the developmentally ventral (anterior) and dorsal (posterior) muscle groups.

Cords

The anterior divisions of the superior and middle trunks unite to form the **lateral cord.** Here is found the **lateral pectoral nerve** (C5-C7), a branch of the lateral cord. The anterior division from the inferior trunk becomes the **medial cord.** Three nerves arise from this cord: the **medial pectoral nerve** (C8-T1), the **medial cutaneous nerve of the arm** (T1), and the **medial cutaneous nerve of the forearm** (C8-T1). The posterior divisions of all three trunks combine to form the **posterior cord.** From the posterior cord arises the **upper subscapular nerve** (C5-C6) to the subscapularis, the **middle subscapular nerve (thoracodorsal nerve,** or nerve to the **latissimus dorsi)** (C6-C8), and the **lower subscapular nerve** (C5-C6) to the teres major, as well as lower fibers of the subscapularis.

Branches

Each anterior cord splits in two. The lateral cord splits into the **musculocutaneous nerve** (C5-C7) and a contribution to the **median nerve.** The medial cord splits into the **ulnar nerve** (C7-T1) and the remainder of the **median nerve** (C5-T1).

TIP The anterior division terminal branches typically form a distinctive M shape, with the median nerve issuing from the center of the M, and the musculocutaneous and ulnar nerves forming the respective limbs of the M. The posterior cord lies posterior to the M shape, deep to the axillary and brachial arteries, in agreement with its posterior division nature.

The posterior cord gives off the upper subscapular (C5), middle subscapular (thoracodorsal) (C7-C8), lower subscapular nerves (C5-C6), and the axillary nerve (C5-C6). The **radial nerve** (C5-T1) innervates the remainder of the muscles of the posterior compartments of the arm and forearm.

Exercises

1. Color in and label in the figure below the cutaneous nerve fields. Indicate the origin of those arising from branches of the brachial plexus and identify their spinal levels. (Contrast this with the dermatomes in this region.)

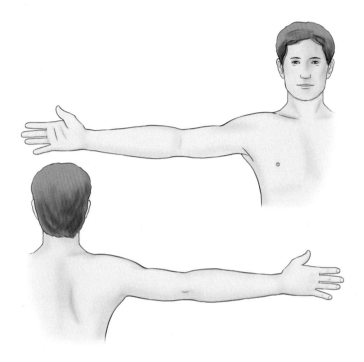

2. Label the components of the brachial plexus in the figure below and indicate the spinal levels represented in each terminal branch. Shade in the posterior (dorsal) division elements.

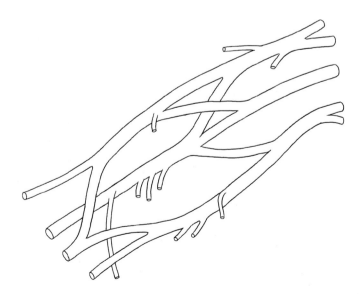

3. Label the branches of the subclavian artery in the figure below.

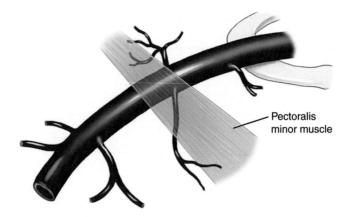

Pectoralis
minor muscle

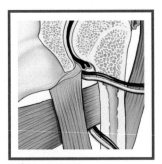

Scapular Region, Shoulder Joint, and Arm

LAB OBJECTIVES

In this lab the musculoskeletal anatomy of the pectoral girdle will be considered further. The muscles arising from the scapula and inserting on the bones of the upper extremity and the anatomy of the shoulder joint are to be examined. On completion of this lab the student will be able to:

- Identify the bony landmarks of the scapula and humerus.
- Identify the muscles of the scapular region and arm innervated by dorsal and ventral divisions of ventral rami of spinal nerves.
- Define the rotator cuff and its function.
- Identify the ligaments and movements of the shoulder joint.

CASE STUDY

The Shoulder Complex: Rude Awakening

Alice is a 52 **y/o** female speech pathologist admitted to the **ER** at 7:00 A.M. complaining of **R** shoulder pain and immobility after she described what sounded like a "clunk" in the shoulder while trying to turn off her alarm clock earlier that morning. Her **PMH** indicates a wide diversity of injuries secondary to being involved in competitive and recreational sports, including water skiing, bicycle racing, running, and cross-country snow skiing. She suffered a frank **dislocation** (total discongruency of bony articulation surfaces) of the same shoulder during a bicycle crash 6 years ago and then **separated** (abrupt stretching or rupture of the acromioclavicular attachments or the coracoclavicular ligamentous attachments, or both) the shoulder 2 years ago while downhill snow skiing.

The **ER** team observes that her shoulder is in a slightly **open-packed position** (allows for greatest joint space), and her arm in a self-splinted or guarded position, with limited **AROM** in flexion, adduction, and external rotation. Palpation reveals **Pt.** tenderness on the anterior deltoid, long head of biceps brachii tendon, and anterior capsule. Before this most recent injury, Alice **c/o** night pain when she sleeps on that side. Her **manual muscle test (MMT)** of the deltoids, rhomboids, and **SITS** musculature (supraspinatus, infraspinatus, teres minor, and subscapularis) revealed weak (3/5) and painful results. **PROM** was also limited and guarded. She had a + **Apprehension Sign** (noted uncomfortable posturing when the shoulder was moved into 90 degrees of abduction and external rotation with posterior-to-anterior pressure at the **GH** joint) and a + **Sulcus Sign** (a dip on the anterior aspect of the GH joint when the arm is placed in abducted manual traction). The x-ray reveals no fracture or displacement of the humerus, clavicle, or scapula. The physician recommends further study with an arthrogram plus orthopedic consult and places the patient on a course of **NSAIDs.** The patient is **D/C** with the **R** shoulder in a sling for joint protection.

Identification of the Anatomy

The shoulder complex is one of the most mobile and least stable regional structures in the body. Hence it has great potential for injury secondary to a very loose capsular structure around the GH joint. Combined with adjacent joints, the shoulder accomplishes a wide array of movements, including proximal direction of the hand to allow for precise manipulations. Furthermore, a host of vital structures, including the axillary neurovascular bundle and the major components of the brachial plexus, are found in intimate contact with the anterior inferior portion of the GH capsule and surrounding musculature. The dissection of the shoulder reveals the differences among the anterior, posterior, inferior, and superior portions of the GH capsule, along with the various ligaments of the supporting acromioclavicular, sternoclavicular, and coracoclavicular joints.

Appreciate the following structures during dissection:

Musculature:
    SITS musculature-rotator cuff—deltoid group
    Pectoral group
    Latissimus dorsi
    Biceps brachii
    Serratus anterior (primary in scapulothoracic
        rhythm motion)
Joint complexes:
    Acromioclavicular, scapulothoracic,
        sternoclavicular, coracoclavicular,
        coracoid process, acromion, clavicle,
        coracoid process
Ligaments:
    Transverse, coracohumeral, trapezoid, conoid,
        acromioclavicular, coracoacromial
Soft tissues:
    Divisions, cords, and branches of the brachial
        plexus, the vascular bundle, components of the
        GH capsule, glenoid labrum

Questions

1. Alice is a patient with a relatively clear presentation as to her signs and symptoms. Given her history and mechanism of injury in this episode, what motions would you think are most problematic for her?
2. What tissue or tissues may be compromised in this patient, leading to her instability?
3. Where is the joint laxity the greatest in patients with this type of abnormality?

Discussion

This patient probably has GH instability secondary to a chronic GH joint laxity in the anterior and inferior

portions of the capsule. Patients with repeated shoulder dislocation, subluxation, or separation often tend to develop shoulder laxity and possible labrum, or rotator cuff tears. Night pain is usually the cardinal symptom of this type of damage, and an arthrogram will generally be used to diagnose the lesion. Patients may have multidirectional instability **(MDI)** or unidirectional instability with the likelihood of a **Bankart lesion** (tear in the anterior capsule). This patient subluxed her shoulder when she turned off her alarm clock in the abducted and externally rotated humeral position. The two positive tests in this patient indicate clear joint laxity. Patients need to be aggressive in strengthening musculature and the capsule around the joint to increase stability or the problem will progressively worsen and require surgical intervention for stabilization. Furthermore, patients with these types of injuries who are sent home in an immobilization sling must be careful to move the shoulder in a pain-tolerable fashion so as to maintain motions and avoid another shoulder abnormality known as *adhesive capsulitis* (frozen shoulder).

Preparation

Identify on the **scapula** (N420, 421; G6.1, 6.31; GY353; C76):
    Borders (margins)
        Median (vertebral)
        Lateral (axillary)
        Superior
    Angles—superior and inferior
    Superior (suprascapular) notch
    Greater scapular notch
    Spine
    Fossae
        Supraspinous
        Infraspinous
        Subscapular
    Acromion process
    Coracoid process
    Glenoid fossa
Identify on the humerus:
    Anatomic neck
    Surgical neck
    Greater tubercle
    Lesser tubercle
    Intertubercular groove
        (bicipital groove)
    Deltoid tuberosity

Dissection

Place the cadaver in a prone position. As necessary, **remove** skin and superficial fascia from the arm and forearm to just below the elbow. **Watch** for the superficial veins and cutaneous nerves (N479; G6.10; GY377; C27, 30, 31).

Identify the basilic vein. In your atlas, **identify** the **superior lateral brachial, inferior lateral brachial, posterior brachial, and medial brachial cutaneous nerves.** *These structures are terminal branches of what nerves?*

Detach the **trapezius** from the **spine of the scapula,** and **reflect** it forward, leaving it attached at the clavicle (N424; G6.29; GY378; C328).

Detach the **deltoid** from the scapular spine and **acromion** of the scapula in a similar manner. **Note** the **axillary nerve** (C5, C6) and the **posterior humeral circumflex artery** emerging from the **quadrangular space** and entering the deltoid (N426, 432; G6.35; GY380; C24, 25). The space is defined superiorly by the capsule of the shoulder joint, laterally by the **surgical neck of the humerus,** medially by the **long head of the triceps,** and inferiorly by the superior border of the **teres major** (Figure 12-1).

Attempt to identify the **subdeltoid bursa** and the **subacromial bursa** (N423; G6.42; GY358; C80).

Clean and **examine** the attachments of the **supraspinatus, infraspinatus,** and **teres minor** muscles (N425; G6.28, 30; GY364, 365; C24, 32). Together with the **subscapularis,** these structures form the **rotator cuff.** The broad flat tendons of these muscles fuse to and reinforce the joint capsule of **glenohumeral joint** anteriorly, superiorly, and posteriorly.

Run your finger along the superior margin of the scapula. *Can you feel the* **suprascapular notch** (N421; G6.31; GY353; C76)? It is bridged by the **suprascapular ligament.** In approximately 20% of the time, the ligament has ossified, forming a *foramen.* Above bony the ligament passes the **suprascapular artery,** and beneath it passes the **suprascapular nerve.**

Make a vertical cut just medial to the notch through the belly of the supraspinatus, and reflect the lateral portion laterally (N426; G6.38; GY366; C25). **Perform** the same procedure with the infraspinatus, and **observe** the suprascapular nerve and artery reaching the infraspinatus muscle through the **greater scapular notch.**

Trace the suprascapular artery and nerve back along the lateral border of the inferior belly of the

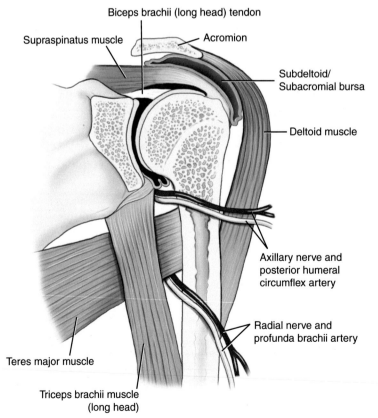

Biceps brachii (long head) tendon

Supraspinatus muscle

Acromion

Subdeltoid/ Subacromial bursa

Deltoid muscle

Axillary nerve and posterior humeral circumflex artery

Radial nerve and profunda brachii artery

Teres major muscle

Triceps brachii muscle (long head)

FIGURE 12-1
Coronal section through the shoulder.

omohyoid muscle until you encounter the **trans-verse cervical artery,** which becomes the **dorsal scapular artery** once past the **superior angle** of the scapula. (Note: *the dorsal scapular artery may arise directly from the subclavian artery.*) It is accompanied by the **dorsal scapular nerve (N427, 429; G6.39; GY366; C25).** Between the teres minor and teres major is the **triangular space.** Deep to this space is the **circumflex scapular artery (N426; G6.38; GY366; C25).**

POSTERIOR MUSCULAR COMPARTMENT OF THE ARM

The **long head of the triceps** passes between the teres major and minor, then attaches to the **infraglenoid tubercle.**

- **Separate** the **lateral and long heads of the triceps** to see the **radial nerve** and the **deep artery of the arm (N432; G6.37, 6.38; GY380; C42, 43)** along the **spiral groove** of the humerus.
- **Section** the lateral head to visualize this neurovascular bundle better.
- **Identify** this groove and the attachments of the lateral and **medial** heads of the triceps on the skeleton **(N421; G6.31; GY373; C76).**
- **Trace** the muscle to its insertion on the **olecranon process** of the **ulna.** The remaining muscle in the posterior compartment is the **anconeus (N444; G6.73; GY378; C54).** Its proximal attachment is on the posterior surface of the **lateral epicondyle,** and it inserts on the lateral surface of the ulna, from the root of the olecranon to the approximately one-third its length.

ANTERIOR MUSCULAR COMPARTMENT OF THE ARM

With the deltoid reflected, **examine** the proximal attachments of the **biceps brachii,** the **short head** with its attachment on the scapular **coracoid** process, and the tendon of the **long head** in the **intertubercular sulcus,** disappearing into the joint capsule of the glenohumeral joint, to attach to the **supraglenoid tubercle** of the scapula. At its distal end, **note** the broad **bicipital aponeurosis** that blends medially in the deep fascia over the forearm flexor muscle group **(N431; G6.33; GY374; C37).** The biceps brachii tendon inserts distally on the **radial tuberosity.**
- **Examine** the remaining two muscles of the anterior compartment: the **coracobrachialis** and the **brachialis.**
- **Trace** the **musculocutaneous nerve** (C5-C7), which pierces the coracobrachialis and travels between the biceps and the brachialis.

GLENOHUMERAL JOINT

- **Review** the osseoligamentous anatomy of the glenohumeral joint in your atlas **(N423; G6.42; GY36; C80, 81).**
- **Reflect** the infraspinatus, which should already be cut laterally, and **separate** it from the joint capsule. **Perform** the same for the teres minor.
- **Cut** a square window from the posterior aspect of the joint capsule.
- **Using** a hammer and osteotome, **remove** the head of the humerus, taking care to place the cut within the joint capsule (Figure 12-2).

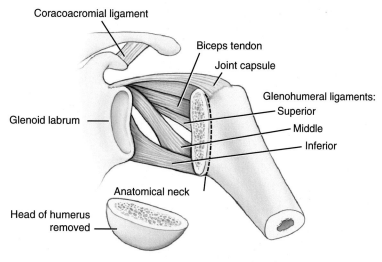

FIGURE 12-2
Posterior view of the interior of the shoulder joint capsule with the humeral head removed, affording a view of the glenohumeral ligaments.

Wash out the joint cavity and attempt to identify the following:

Tendon of the biceps brachii long head. Note that it passes through the joint capsule but lies without the synovial membrane.

Superior GH ligament. Found just below and parallel to the tendon of the biceps brachii long head.

Middle GH ligament. Oriented obliquely.

Inferior GH ligament. Flanks anterior glenoid margin.

TIP Note that the glenohumeral ligaments are thickenings of the joint capsule and may not have discrete borders that can easily be observed.

*What is the relationship of the **coracoacromial ligament** to the head of the humerus?* Note also that the **coracoacromial arch** prevents upward dislocation of the humerus.

Exercises

1. On the diagram of scapula, sketch and label all muscle attachments.

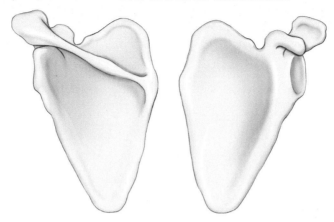

2. In this lateral view of a semitransparent humerus, label the tendons of the rotator cuff, and describe how you would test for weakness in each muscle.

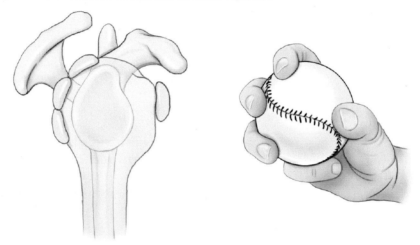

3. Describe the anatomic basis for the high proportion of *anterior* dislocations of the shoulder. In what activities might such an injury occur?

Elbow and Forearm

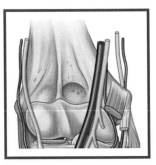

LAB OBJECTIVES

In this lab the structures crossing the elbow joint will be considered further. The topographic anatomy of the cubital fossa will be examined. The muscles of the forearm will be deciphered. On completion of this lab the student should be able to:

- Identify the bony landmarks of the distal humerus, proximal radius, and ulna.
- Identify the muscles of the forearm; their attachments; their innervations by branches of the radial, median, or ulnar nerves; and their actions.
- Identify the ligaments and describe movements of the elbow joint.

CASE STUDY

Precision Hand Function Needed

During an ergonomics presentation to a group of dental hygienists, an **OT** addresses the issue of appropriate body mechanics from the 11:00 to 2:00 o'clock positions when hygienists work with patients in the dental operatory. A hygienist asks a question concerning numbness and tingling in his dominant hand after he has treated several patients and whether this has anything to do with positioning his body when treating the patient. The **OT** asks the hygienist to stop in at the clinic afterward for an examination, which reveals the following. The patient is a 28 **y/o** right hand dominant male with **c/o** of numbness, pain (3/10), and weakness in the right hand after a full day of work as a dental hygienist. His **PMH** is unremarkable other than a medial epicondylar fracture when he was 20 **y/o.** He is moderately active by walking and playing tennis twice a week with friends. He is concerned about being unable to control his oral cleaning instruments and drops them on occasion, which increases his treatment time with the patients. The OT examination reveals **B upper quarter screen (UQS)** is normal with the exception of a slight decrease in the **R** hand intrinsic musculature strength and slight decrease in sensation in the fourth and fifth fingers. The patient exhibits a + **Tinel's sign** (tapping over a superficial nerve gives rise to pain in the nerve distribution) over the radial and median nerves and a + **Upper Limb Tension Test (ULTT),** (progressive manual tension in the upper extremity to provoke traction on various nerve from the brachial plexus). Also noted is considerable muscle hypertrophy of the **R** forearm. The patient suggests that the pain goes away in the evening and with rest.

Identification of the Anatomy

The elbow complex is unique in its joint architecture because it has three different joints performing specialized functions. The radioulnar, radiohumeral, and ulnohumeral act in concert to provide some aspects of elbow flexion and extension, as well as forearm pronation and supination. Careful dissection of the space anterior to the elbow, the cubital fossa, will give exposure to the various structures crossing this area, including the neurovascular bundle, common extrinsic muscles, some of which are biarticulate, and nerves that innervate the hand. Clinicians use this area to gain vital diagnostic information, including **BP,** blood samples, electromyographic **(EMG)** data, and nerve conduction study **(NCS)**.

Appreciate the following structures during dissection:

Musculature/nerves:
    Common flexor and extensor tendons, both superficial and deep groups, with associated nerves and vessels (radial, median and ulnar nerves, radial and ulnar arteries and veins)
Joint complex:
    Radial head, radial tuberosity, humeroradial joint, radioulnar joint, and ulnohumeral joint, olecranon process/fossa, coronoid process, trochlear, trochlear notch, ulnar groove
Ligaments:
    Annular ligament, medial and lateral collateral ligaments, interosseous membrane
Soft tissue/vessels:
    Radial, ulnar, brachial and brachii profundi arteries, median cubital and basilic veins, bicipital aponeurosis

Questions

1. The signs and symptoms of the patient would indicate what nerve involvement? Why?
2. Can you postulate a mechanism for causing the signs and symptoms in this patient?

Discussion

Regardless of the region of the body, nerve entrapment syndromes are commonplace, especially with abnormal use patterns such as those seen in different types of occupations. Only approximately 1 kg of pressure is needed to cause nerve damage, and this pressure can be brought on by increased fluid content in and around a nerve, abnormal bony morphology, tight musculature, tight synovial sheaths, or several other factors. Normally, this compression results in ischemia of the nerve, leading to pain, numbness, tingling, and eventual lose of function. In this case, the patient has an entrapment of the ulnar nerve at the elbow. This entrapment might have occurred secondarily to faulty and constant flexed elbow posture during work, a bony abnormality at the elbow as a result of his past medial epicondylar fractures, or simple overuse. The ulnar nerve is involved because of the noted sensory distribution deficits and partial motor

weakness into the hand. Clear diagnosis should involve an **NCS** and radiographs.

Preparation

Identify on the **humerus** (N436; G6.49; GY372; C84, 87):
    Capitulum
    Trochlea
    Medial and lateral epicondyles
    Medial and lateral supracondylar ridges
    Coronoid fossa
    Olecranon fossa

Identify on the **radius:**
    Head
    Neck
    Tuberosity

Identify on the **ulna:**
    Olecranon process
    Trochlear notch
    Coronoid process
    Radial notch
    Tuberosity

Dissection

Place the cadaver in a supine position. As necessary, **remove** skin and superficial fascia from the forearm to the wrist.

Watch for the superficial veins and cutaneous nerves (N480; G6.6, 6.10; GY423-425; C44, 45). **Note** the highly variable tributaries of the **basilic** and **cephalic veins,** which are bridged across the cubital fossa by the **median cubital vein.**

Define the cutaneous nerve fields of the **medial, lateral,** and **posterior cutaneous nerves of the forearm (antebrachium)** (N481; G6.6; GY424, 425; C26). *These cutaneous nerve fields are terminal branches of what nerves?*

The triangular area anterior to the elbow joint is called the **cubital fossa** (N446; G6.45; GY390; C46). The triangle is bounded by the **pronator teres, brachioradialis,** and a line between the epicondyles. The principal contents of the fossa are the **bicipital tendon,** the **brachial artery,** and **m**edian nerve, which can be remembered by the acronym **BAM.** Lateral to the bicipital tendon is the **lateral cutaneous nerve of the forearm,** the terminal branch of the musculocutaneous nerve.

The brachial artery divides into the **radial** and **ulnar arteries (N447; G6.45; GY390; C47).** The radial artery passes superficial to the pronator teres and then travels deep to the brachioradialis. The ulnar artery gives off the **common interosseus artery** before passing deep to the pronator teres then travels with the ulnar nerve deep to the **flexor carpi ulnaris.**

Examine a diagram of the arterial anastomoses around the elbow **(N434; G6.7; GY376; C17).**

Identify as many of these collateral branches as you can.

ANTERIOR (FLEXOR) COMPARTMENT

As needed, **reflect** the bicipital aponeurosis. **Note** that many of the flexors of the forearm arise from the medial epicondyle of the humerus from a common flexor tendon **(N450; G6.59; GY396; [C47]).**

Carefully clean away the deep fascia, and **separate** each muscle belly of the flexor compartment.

Determine the origin, insertion, and action of each muscle belly, and record in the table in Exercise 1 (insertions distal to the wrist will be confirmed in the subsequent lab). They are innervated by branches of the median nerve, except for the flexor carpi ulnaris (C7-C8) and the ulnar bellies of the flexor digitorum profundus (C8-T1), which receive innervation from the ulnar nerve.

Identify the *superficial layer* **(N446, 442; G6.57, 6.58; GY398; C46)** of the flexor compartment moving from lateral to medial:

>   **Pronator teres (C6-C7)**
>   **Flexor carpi radialis (C6-C7)**
>   **Palmaris longus (C7-C8) (absent in 10%)**
>   **Flexor carpi ulnaris (C7-C8)**

Note the pattern of organization: the two flexors of the wrist flank palmaris longus and the flexors of the digits.

Trace the ulnar nerve as it passes posterior to the medial epicondyle and travels deep to the flexor carpi ulnaris.

Identify the *intermediate layer* **(N447, 443; G6.58; Gy399; C47):**

>   Flexor digitorum superficialis (C7-T1)

Section the radial head of the flexor digitorum superficialis.

Observe the median nerve as it travels deep to this muscle. **Identify** the **anterior interosseus nerve** and **artery.**

Identify the *deep layer* **(N448, 443; G6.59, 6.60; GY399, 400; C46):**

>   **Flexor policis longus (C8-T1)**
>   **Flexor digitorum profundus (C8-T1)**
>   **Pronator quadratus (C8-T1)**

Note that the tendon to the index finger is a nearly separate muscle belly, giving this finger much independence of action in flexion (Figure 13-1).

POSTERIOR (EXTENSOR) COMPARTMENT

Notice that the majority of the extensor muscles of the forearm arise from the lateral epicondyle of the humerus by means of a common extensor compartment. The basic pattern is repeated: Extensors of the wrist flank the extensors of the digits. They are innervated by branches of the **radial nerve.**

Identify the *superficial layer* **(N444, 441; G6.73; GY401):**
>   Brachioradialis (C5-C7)
>   Extensor carpi radialis longus and brevis (C6-C7)
>   Extensor digitorum (communis) (C7-C8)
>   Extensor digiti minimi (C7-C8)
>   Extensor carpi ulnaris (C7-C8)

The brachioradialis is considered with the extensors because it is also innervated by the radial nerve. However, it assists in flexion of the elbow, especially when the forearm is pronated.

Find the **radial nerve** where it lies anterior to the lateral epicondyle, between the brachialis and the brachioradialis.

Observe it split into the superficial and deep branches. The **superficial branch of the radial nerve** travels under the brachioradials and ends in the dorsum of the hand. The deep branch passes through the supinator.

Identify the *deep layer* **(N445, 441; G6.74; GY402, 403; C52, 53):**
>   Abductor pollicis longus (C7-C8)
>   Extensor pollicis brevis (C7-C8)
>   Extensor pollicis longus (C7-C8)
>   Extensor indicis (C7-C8)

Deep to the extensor digitorum, **locate** the **posterior interosseus artery** as it emerges from beneath the supinator and the **deep branch of the radial nerve** as it pierces the supinator (Figure 13-2).

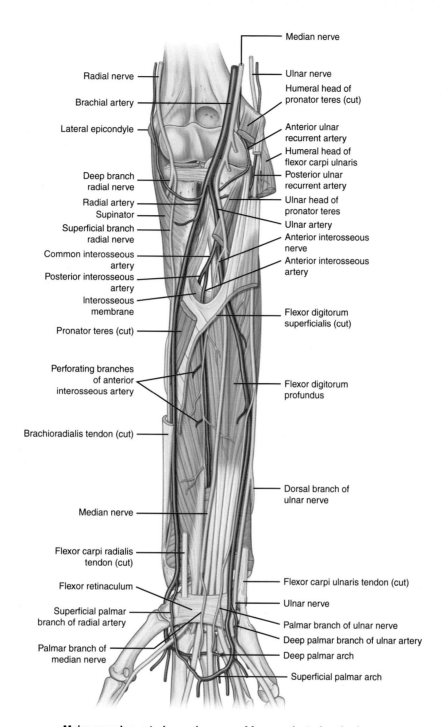

Radial nerve

Brachial artery

Lateral epicondyle

Deep branch
radial nerve

Radial artery

Supinator

Superficial branch
radial nerve

Common interosseous
artery

Posterior interosseous
artery

Interosseous
membrane

Pronator teres (cut)

Perforating branches
of anterior
interosseous artery

Brachioradialis tendon (cut)

Median nerve

Flexor carpi radialis
tendon (cut)

Flexor retinaculum

Superficial palmar
branch of radial artery

Palmar branch of
median nerve

Median nerve

Ulnar nerve

Humeral head of
pronator teres (cut)

Anterior ulnar
recurrent artery

Humeral head of
flexor carpi ulnaris

Posterior ulnar
recurrent artery

Ulnar head of
pronator teres

Ulnar artery

Anterior interosseous
nerve

Anterior interosseous
artery

Flexor digitorum
superficialis (cut)

Flexor digitorum
profundus

Dorsal branch of
ulnar nerve

Flexor carpi ulnaris tendon (cut)

Ulnar nerve

Palmar branch of ulnar nerve

Deep palmar branch of ulnar artery

Deep palmar arch

Superficial palmar arch

Major muscles, arteries and nerves of forearm (anterior view)

FIGURE 13-1

Major muscles, arteries and nerves of the anterior compartment of the forearm. (From Drake, R et al: *Gray's Atlas of Anatomy,1e*, Philadelphia, 2008, Churchill Livingstone.)

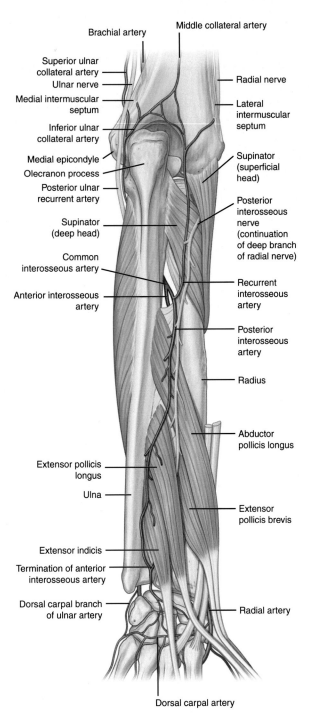

Brachial artery

Middle collateral artery

Superior ulnar collateral artery

Ulnar nerve

Medial intermuscular septum

Inferior ulnar collateral artery

Medial epicondyle

Olecranon process

Posterior ulnar recurrent artery

Supinator (deep head)

Common interosseous artery

Anterior interosseous artery

Extensor pollicis longus

Ulna

Extensor indicis

Termination of anterior interosseous artery

Dorsal carpal branch of ulnar artery

Radial nerve

Lateral intermuscular septum

Supinator (superficial head)

Posterior interosseous nerve (continuation of deep branch of radial nerve)

Recurrent interosseous artery

Posterior interosseous artery

Radius

Abductor pollicis longus

Extensor pollicis brevis

Radial artery

Dorsal carpal artery

Major muscles, arteries and nerves in the deep posterior compartment of forearm

FIGURE 13-2

Major muscles, arteries and nerves of the deep posterior compartment of the forearm. (From Drake, R et al: *Gray's Atlas of Anatomy,1e*, Philadelphia, 2008, Churchill Livingstone.)

Elbow Joint

Review the osseoligamentous anatomy of the elbow joint in your atlas (**N438; G6.51-54; GY388, 389; C87, 88**).

As necessary, **detach** the soft tissue from the elbow joint capsule.

Identify the ulnar collateral ligament, which consists of a strong anterior cord, a weaker posterior fanlike portion, and a transverse band.

On the lateral side, **expose** the radial collateral ligament. **Note** that it attaches to the annular ligament rather than to the radius itself. *Why?* The annular ligament encircles the head of the radius. *What are its attachments on the ulna?*

Open the capsule anteriorly by cutting transversely between the collateral ligaments. **Explore** the extent of the capsule.

Clinical Note

Tissue Loading Forces

All biologic tissue has characteristics that are *rate dependent,* giving them different strengths, depending on forces and rates of loading. A tendon can actually be stronger than a bone when it is loaded slowly, resulting in an *avulsion* of the bone. The mechanism that allows for this type of fracture is related to the Sharpey fibers located in the transition of the tendon of a muscle into the periosteum of the bone Sharpey's fibers penetrate and are embedded in the bony matrix deep to the periosteum. The transition of collagen fibers allows the tendon to become continuous with the periosteum over and *fan out* over the bone. Avulsions are not uncommon at the radial tuberosity, lesser trochanter, and calcaneus in response to the large tension of their respective tendon attachments.

Exercises

1. Fill in the accompanying table, identifying the attachments and deducing the actions of the muscles of the forearm.

Muscle	Origin	Insertion	Action

2. What are the axes of rotation found in the elbow joints?

3. When you hit your *funny bone,* what anatomic structure is really involved? What bony feature is associated?

Wrist and Hand

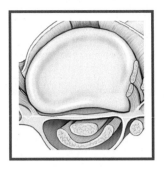

CASE STUDY

Wrist Pain: The Court Reporter

Jane is a 42 **y/o** court reporter for several attorneys. She is responsible for recording the depositions of plaintiffs, defendants, and expert witnesses. She works 3 days a week for approximately 4 to 6 hours a day. For the last 6 months, she experienced pain in both hands; specifically at the **MCP** joints and the wrist of her right hand during and after taking recordings. She describes the pain as tolerable but notes that it has become intermittently worse over the last few months. She states that she feels a little swelling over the back **(dorsum)** and front **(volar)** surface of the wrist. In addition, she suggests that the wrists feel a bit "boggy" at night. She has also noticed a nodule on her proximal interphalangeal **(PIP)** joint of the third finger. She states her hand hurts and is stiff more in the mornings but that the pain and stiffness subside during the day until she begins work. She indicates that she has had an ergonomic analysis performed on her workstation by an **OT**, but this did not seem to alter her symptoms. She also indicates that she has felt a bit fatigued, and this is highly unusual for her, given her active recreational lifestyle.

Identification of the Anatomy

The dissection of the wrist and hand can be tedious. However, if performed with care, the anatomy revealed gives the student a clear understanding of the specific function of these structures in daily activities. As with other dissections, you need to be delicate with the scalpel and emphasize more blunt techniques when dissecting through the palmer and dorsal aspects of both the wrist and the hand to identify the deep structures. Take careful note of the structure of the carpal tunnel and its contents and the various annular and cruciate *pulleys* of the hand. These pulleys and the tendons they house are intricately related to some of the more common degenerative and traumatic pathologic conditions seen in the hand and wrist.

Appreciate the following structures during dissection:

>   Contents of the carpal tunnel
>   Ulnar and median nerves
>   Examination of the MCP, PIP, and distal
>   interphalangeal (DIP) joints of the fingers
>   Carpal bone grouping
>   Extensor hood mechanism
>   Median and ulnar nerves and arteries
>   Flexor and extensor retinaculae

Questions

1. When tissues are painful and enlarged, what does this usually indicate?
2. All synovial joints are harbors for the work of both internal and external forces that may alter function and bring on degeneration and possibly trauma. What are some diseases that alter joint function?
3. What are the differences between osteoarthritis and rheumatoid arthritis?

Discussion

In this case, Jane exhibits some of the classic signs and symptoms of rheumatoid arthritis **(RA)**. The disease onset occurs in young to middle-age women, with inherited traits. This disease is one of inflammation and with an autoimmune cause. Although the precise origin of RA is unknown, it clearly involves the proliferation of synovium in the joints and the tendons and sheaths around the joints. This condition is called **tenosynovitis.** The nodes present in the disease are commonly called **Bouchard's nodes**, which form on the **PIP. Heberden's nodes** also form at the DIP but are most common in **osteoarthritis.** The swelling is caused by inflammation and seems to be intermittent in nature. Approximately 15% of patients with RA go into full remission, and 10% progress to advanced stages regardless of treatment. Late stages of progressive disease can render the hands and other joints useless because major deformities in the fingers and wrists can rupture tendons and ligaments and destroy the joints. Additionally, other bodily systems can be affected, leading to major systemic complications. Patients need to be referred to other members of the health care team to ensure early treatment and continued medical management of the condition.

Preparation

Identify on the distal **ulna** and **radius** (N452; G6.56, 6.72; GY392; C90, 91):

Ulnar styloid process
Radial styloid process
Dorsal tubercle of the radius
Identify the individual **carpals** (N452; G6.80; GY392; C90, 91). They lie in two rows of four.
>   Beginning on the radial side of the proximal row we find:
>   **Scaphoid**
>   **Lunate**
>   **Triquetrium**
>   **Pisiform**
>   The distal row consists of:
>   **Trapezium**
>   **Trapezoid**
>   **Capitate**
>   **Hamate**

TIP One way to remember them in this order is to create a silly saying such as:

"Some leprechauns tote pots that they couldn't hide."

You can create your own.

A good exercise to familiarize yourself with the individual carpals is to identify distinguishing features on the individual disarticulated carpals. Here are some suggestions:

Scaphoid	Peanut shaped
Lunate	Crescent moon shaped
Triquetrum	Bears a slightly raised mesa-shaped articular surface for the pisiform
Pisiform	Pea-shaped
Trapezium	Sellar joint; ridge for the transverse carpal ligament
Trapezoid	Angular; peaked roof–shaped distal ridge
Capitate	Chess pawn-shaped
Hamate	Hook for attachment of the transverse carpal ligament

Identify on the **metacarpals** and **phalanges** (N456; G6.80; GY394; C90):

Base
Shaft
Head

Anatomic Overview

The bulk of the muscles responsible for movements of the fingers lie in the forearms (i.e., extrinsic muscles). Their distal attachments are achieved by long tendons of insertion that span multiple joints. These tendons are formed from **dense, regular connective tissue.** The regular arrangement of the connective tissue is in response to tension exerted in one direction. Each tendon is surrounded by loose, fibrous connective tissue, the tendon sheath, or **paratendineum** (Figure 14-1). Its inner surface, which lies in contact with the tendon, is called the **epitendineum.** Bundles of collagen fibers are clustered in a cable-like fashion and surrounded by **endotendineum,** which contains blood vessels and nerves, forming the primary fascicles. When not stretched, the primary fascicles have a wavy appearance (crimp) in longitudinal section. This arrangement allows the tendon to give slightly when a contraction of the muscle is initiated. Molecular collagen can be stretched only 4% to 5% of its length and has a high tensile strength (500-1000 kg/cm^2). Therefore tendons have a greater resistance to rupture than muscles. The tendon cells are fibrocytes and are compressed between bundles of collagen fibers, creating winglike cytoplasmic processes.

Dissection

Review the cutaneous innervation of the hand (N472; G6.75; GY424, 425; C26).

Remove the remaining skin and superficial fascia from the hand and fingers. Take care over the palm, observing the firm attachment of the palmar superficial fascia to the underlying **palmar aponeurosis** (N459; G6.63, 6.65; GY409; CC62).

Compare the mobility of the skin of your own palm to the skin on the dorsum of your hand. As you skin the palm, take care to observe the **palmaris brevis** muscle, the fibers of which run transversely from the palmar aponeurosis in an ulnar direction (N459; G6.63; GY409; C64). Pressing on the pisiform will elicit a contraction of the palmaris brevis and produce wrinkles over the ulnar side of the palm. Forcefully abducting the fifth digit will produce the same result. On the radial side of the palm, **watch** for the **recurrent branch of the median nerve.** On the palmar surface of the wrist and hand, **note** the tendon of the **palmaris longus** running into the **palmar aponeurosis.**

Clench your fist tightly, and **observe** the prominent tendons crossing your ventral wrist (G6.63; GY409). The more medial and slightly more superficial is the palmaris longus tendon.

Clean and **trace** the fibers of the palmar aponeurosis. Some fibers extend into the digits; some encircle the long flexor tendons and then attach to the deep transverse metacarpal ligament. **Notice** the chicken-drumstick–shaped cluster of muscles on either side of the palm. These muscles are the **thenar** (thumb-side) and **hypothenar** (pinky-side) **eminences.**

Clean and **separate** the following muscles (N460; G6.67; GY410; C65):

Thenar eminence:
  Abductor pollicis brevis (C8-T1)
  Flexor pollicis brevis (C8-T1)
    Note that this superficial pair of muscles crosses the metacarpophalangeal (MCP) joint to insert on the base of the proximal phalanx.
  Opponens pollicis (C8-T1)
    Section the mid-belly, and reflect the thenar eminence to reveal the opponens pollicis. Note that this deeper muscle inserts along the length of the metacarpal shaft.

Hypothenar eminence:
  Abductor digiti minimi (C8-T1)
  Flexor digiti minimi brevis (C8-T1)
    These muscles exhibit an arrangement very similar to their counterparts at the pollex.
  Opponens digiti minimi (C8-T1)
    Section and reflect the muscles of the hypothenar eminence to reveal the opponens digiti minimi.

Reflect the palmar aponeurosis distally.

Examine the **transverse carpal ligament (flexor retinaculum)** (N443; G6.62; C66). It spans the arch of the combined carpus, attached to the **hook of the hamate,** pisiform, **tubercle of the trapezium,** and **tubercle of the scaphoid,** forming an osseoligamentous **carpal tunnel** (N461; G6.68; GY411; C67). The ligament is approximately the size of standard postage stamp situated just distal to the most distal flexion crease in the skin over the ventral wrist.

Carefully transect the ligament without disturbing the structures deep to it. Within the tunnel are the tendons of the flexor digitorum superficialis and profundus. A common **synovial sheath,** also known as the **ulnar bursa,** encompasses these tendons (N462, 463; G6.68; GY410; C72, 73).

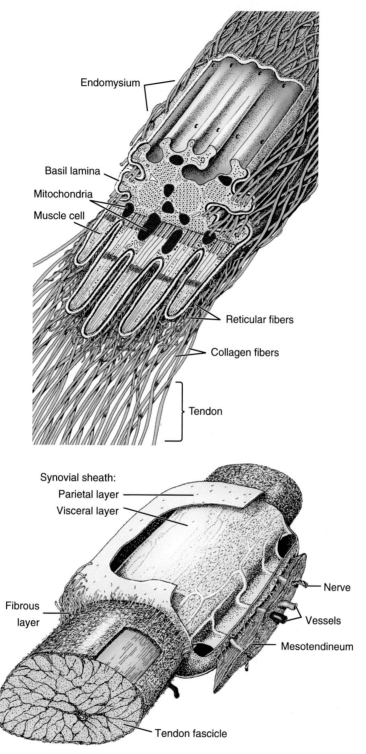

FIGURE 14-1
Structural histology of the tendon and the myotendinal junction. (*Modified from Krstic RV: General histology of the mammal, Berlin, 1984, Springer-Verlag.*)

TIP Using a hypodermic needle (if available), **inject** some water colored with blue food coloring into the synovial sheath to make it more visible. If the sheath has not been nicked, the dye will spread throughout its extent.

Separate within the tunnel the tendon of the flexor pollicis longus within its synovial sheath, the **radial bursa.**

Identify the **median nerve** within the tunnel. It is the structure most susceptible to compression within the confines of the carpal tunnel.

Trace the flexor tendons into the digits. **Examine** the **annular and cruciform parts of the fibrous flexor sheaths** (N463; G6.68; GY410; C72). These structures encircle the digital synovial sheaths surrounding the flexor tendons. Open one or two of the sheaths, and examine the tendons.

Section the fleshy bellies of the **flexor digitorum superficialis** muscle, and pull the tendons distally.

Separate them from the tendons of the **flexor digitorum profundus.**

Examine their insertions. *How does the tendon of the flexor digitorum superficialis achieve a more proximal attachment than the tendon of the flexor digitorum profundus?*

Clinical Note

Carpal tunnel syndrome (CTS)

People who perform repetitive activities with their hands, such as assembly line workers, meat packers, typists, tailors, and so forth, may experience pain and hypothesia over the radial side of the hand and weakness of grip between the thumb and index finger. The repeated flexion of the fingers during cyclic activities may cause inflammation of the synovial sheaths surrounding the flexor tendons housed in the carpal tunnel. Increased fluid pressure within the bursa compresses the contents of the carpal tunnel, including the median nerve, compromising its sensory and motor functions distal to the wrist. Interestingly, signs and symptoms of CTS can also be caused by pregnancy and disorders involving the endocrine system, which may alter fluid retention. Review the distribution of the median nerve (N458; G6.65). Progressive loss of strength in the thumb may necessitate a carpal tunnel release, a surgical division of the flexor retinaculum.

Identify the **vincula** (N464; G6.69; GY419; C67), which are sleeves of mesothelium encompassing the neurovascular bundles that supply the tendon. Where the **annular fibrous flexor sheaths** fuse with the anterior surface of the **MCP** and **interphalangeal (IP) joints,** they form the **palmar plates** (Figure 14-2).

Locate the **lumbricals** arising from the flexor digitorum profundus tendons (N463; G6.68; GY411; C68). They pass ventral to the **deep transverse metacarpal ligaments** (N458; G6.71; GY415; C92, 93) to insert in the **extensor expansion.** The deep transverse metacarpal ligaments serve to prevent spreading of the metacarpal heads.

Section the muscle bellies of the flexor digitorum profundus in the forearm, and **reflect** them distally, exposing the **palmar and hypothenar spaces** (N4462, 463; G6.64; C72).

Examine the deep branches of the ulnar nerve and artery (N465; G6.73, 6.74; GY415).

Examine and reflect the **adductor pollicis.**

Locate the **sesamoid bones** in the tendous of the **flexor pollicis brevis.**

Identify the **palmar interossei.** *To which digits do they insert?* Their tendons pass dorsal to deep transverse metacarpal ligament.

TIP Section the deep transverse metacarpal ligament between digits three and four to facilitate separating the digits to examine the attachments of the interossei.

Why is flexing the fourth and fifth **carpometacarpal joints** possible? Consult a hand skeleton.

The four tendons of the **extensor digitorum (communis)** (C7-C8) cross the wrist and fan out toward the respective metacarpal heads. Transverse intertendinous fibers unite the tendons and limit their independent action (N470; G6.79; C62). Over the metatarsophalangeal joints, the tendons are anchored to the **palmar plate** (N464; G6.76; GY419; C67) by **transverse laminae,** forming an **extensor hood.** The extensor tendon trifurcates over the proximal phalanx.

Identify the **central band.** *Where does it insert?*

Identify the two **lateral bands,** which ultimately unite to form the so-called **terminal tendon.** *Where does it insert?* The lateral bands are joined by tendinous fibers from the lumbricals and the dorsal

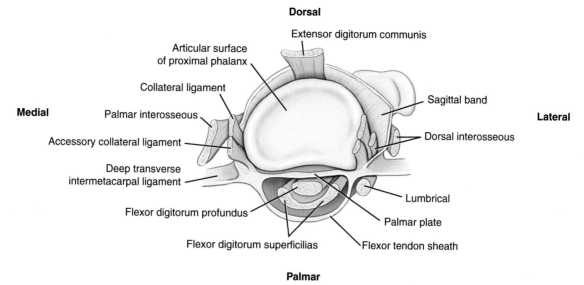

FIGURE 14-2

Proximal view of the base of the proximal phalanx of the left index finger.

interossei to form a complex over the back of the digit called the **extensor expansion** (or **dorsal aponeurosis**).

Locate a fibrous band that arises from the flexor sheath at the proximal phalanx and courses obliquely across the middle phalanx to join the extensor expansion. This fibrous band is the **retinacular ligament (G.6.77)**.

The first and fifth digits are afforded greater independence of movement by the presence of separate extensor muscle bellies.

Locate the superficial **extensor digiti minimi (C7-C8)** muscle and the deeper **extensor indicis (C7-C8)**. Their tendons fuse with those of the extensor digitorum to the second and fifth digits.

Identify the **dorsal interossei (C8-T1) (N465; G6.73; GY420; C68)**. *Remember, they are part of the ventral (anterior) compartment of the hand*, but they lie dorsal to the palmar interossei. **Note** the bipennate architecture of their bellies, which arise from adjacent metacarpal shafts. **Trace** their tendons distally to their insertions on the bases of the

proximal phalanges. **Note** that portions of the tendon blend into the extensor expansion.

Trace and **identify** the insertions of the tendons of the **extensor pollicis longus** and **brevis (C7-C8)** and the **abductor pollicis longus (C7-C8) (N467; G6.78; GY422; C62)** if not already completed. When the thumb is extended, a depression is often noticeable between these two sets of tendons, called the anatomic snuffbox. Note the course of the **radial artery** under the anatomic snuffbox and through the gap between the heads of the first dorsal interosseus.

With the index finger extended, **adduct** the extended pollex. The resulting bulge is the first dorsal interosseus.

Reflect the extensor expansion between the third and fourth digits, and **cut** the extensor hood to reveal the joint capsule **(N458; G6.87; GY421; C92, 93)**.

Locate the **collateral ligament,** an obliquely running band of fibers reinforcing the sides of the MCP joint capsule. With the joint extended, the ligament is slack. With the joint flexed, this ligament is taut.

Demonstrate the reduced range of abduction-adduction in your own MCP joint in flexion versus extension.

Exercises

1. Indicate in the figure below the sensory distributions of the radial, median, and ulnar nerves.

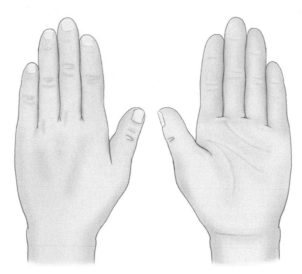

2. Consider the layered organization of the hand as seen in cross-section through the palm. Identify and label the indicated structures on the figure below.

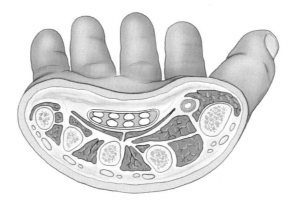

3. Place your hand palm down on a tabletop with the middle digit flexed under the palm. Now attempt to raise each remaining finger from the surface of the table. Are you successful or not? Why?

4. Why is flexing the fourth and fifth carpometacarpal joints possible? Consult a hand skeleton.

5. On the radiograph of the wrist below, identify the individual carpals.

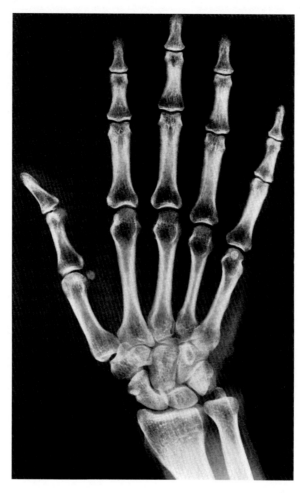

From Wicke L: *Atlas of radiologic anatomy,* ed 7, Munich, 2001. Urban & Fischer.

Posterior Body Wall

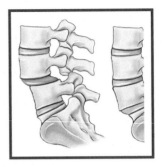

LAB OBJECTIVES

In this lab the musculoskeletal elements comprising the posterior abdominal body wall are considered. The branches of the lumbosacral plexus of nerves are examined and identified. On completing this exploration the student should be able to:

- Describe the relationship of the diaphragm, psoas, and quadratus lumborum to the posterior abdominal body wall.
- Discuss the organization and distribution of the lumbosacral plexus.
- Trace the terminal branches of the abdominal aorta and the tributaries of the inferior vena cava.
- Describe the anatomy of the intervertebral disc, and discuss the reasons for incidence of disc herniation in the lumbar region.

CASE STUDY

The Flexible Back

A 17 **y/o** boy comes to the **ER** after a pick-up basketball game in which he indicates he extended his back while landing inappropriately after a jump shot. The **PA** takes his history, which indicates that he has had intermittent **LBP** during high school physical education class and notices it more when he is standing and improves when he is sitting and is nonexistent in supine with his back flat. He denies **B radicular** symptoms. His **lower quarter screen (LQS)** is negative, with the exception of frank pain when testing the hip flexor musculature. Marked tenderness is noted when palpating and gliding the L5 spinous process anteriorly while the patient is in the prone position. The patient is **D/C** from the **ER** with an **Rx** for ibuprofen and told to place ice on the low back and rest for the next 24 hours.

Identification of the Anatomy

The lumbar region of the vertebral column is by far the most prominent region compromised by inappropriate activity, sports, and overall deconditioned state. Two thirds of the body mass rests on the lower vertebrae in the lumbar region, which is acted on by compression, tension, and shear forces coming from normal motions of the body. The lumbar vertebra and discs are designed to negotiate large loads but need to be stabilized by the surrounding soft tissues and the stability of the various articulation surfaces on each vertebra, as well as the purchase on the sacrum. The proper alignments of the vertebrae are essential during activities to avoid inappropriate joint surface motion **(arthrokinematics)** and bone segment motion **(osteokinematics).**

Appreciate the following structures during dissection:

Bony vertebrae:

  Transitional region from the T12-L1 segment

**Degenerative
spondylolisthesis**

**Isthmic
spondylolisthesis**

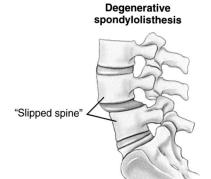
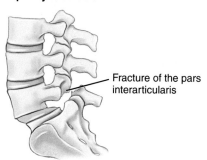

"Slipped spine"

Fracture of the pars
interarticularis

Lumbar inferior and superior facet joint orientation
Pars interarticularis, pedicles, laminae
Central canal
Bony pelvis:
  Ilium, ischium, pubis
  Pelvic inlet and pelvic outlet
Vessels:
  Abdominal aorta and branches
  Inferior vena cava and tributaries
Ligaments and muscles:
  Anterior longitudinal ligament
  Ligaments, iliolumbar
  Inguinal canal and ring
  Psoas major quadratus lumborum

Questions

1. What structures would be provoked or shifted with placing the hip flexors on tension?
2. Can an explanation be found for the onset of this condition?

Discussion

The description and history of this patient are consistent with a condition called **spondylolisthesis.** This condition is the result of one vertebra slipping (subluxation) on another. The lumbar vertebrae and associated transverse processes are the common origin of the psoas muscle, which flexes the hip or the trunk during strength screening. The anterior attachments on the vertebra pull it forward increasing the shear force on those segments and hence causing pain. The same is true when the spinous process of L5 is palpated as it is pressed forward, causing pain in this patient. The patient experiences pain when he stands because of increased weight bearing and shear on that segment. Spondylolisthesis occurs as a result of a congenital deformity, elongation, or a **B** fracture of the pars interarticularis, which allows for the movement of one vertebra on another because facet joints no

longer support the shear or compression moments of the vertebra above. This condition is sometimes called the *Scotty Dog* fracture from the appearance in the oblique view of an x-ray. This condition usually occurs at the L5-S1 levels but can occur at other levels. In older patients, spondylolisthesis may occur caused by degenerative changes in the vertebra. Sometimes, surgical fusion is recommended because the subluxation is so great that it compromises the cauda equina. Conservative treatment invoking strengthening, proper body mechanics, and rest from activity are usually successful in resolving the condition. A similar condition called **spondylolysis** also involves the same defect, but it is unilateral and subluxation does not occur.

Preparation

On an articulated skeleton (N248; G4.22; GY202; C265, 266), identify the following:
  Lumbar vertebrae, transverse processes
  Sacrum
  Auricular surface
  Sacral promontory
  Iliac tuberosity
  Ala of the ilium
  Arcuate line of the ilium

Anatomic Overview

The **lumbosacral plexus** is not as accessible as the brachial plexus, but many of its components can be visualized in the posterior abdominal body wall. The lower extremity is an outgrowth of the ventrolateral body wall, and hence its structures are innervated by an outgrowth of ventral rami of spinal nerves. The skin and muscle are derived from L2 through S3 hypaxial dermamyotomes. As in the upper extremity, these dermamyotomes divide into dorsal and ventral limb components during development. Therefore each ventral ramus carries axons that can be classified as dorsal division or ventral division. These axons segregate and interweave between spinal levels. However, the interweaving of L2 though L4 (lumbar plexus) is nearly independent of that of L5 to S1 (sacral plexus) (Figure 15-1). A small bundle running from L4 to L5 connects the two. The product of this union is called the **lumbosacral trunk.**

During development the lower extremity undergoes a rotation that affects the position of its compartments. The developmentally dorsal compartments come to lie to the lateral and anterior aspects of the extremity, whereas the developmentally ventral compartments are medial and posterior (in contrast, the compartments of the upper extremity in anatomical position approximate their developmental relationships). The lumbar plexus produces one dorsal division nerve, the **femoral nerve,** which supplies muscles of the anterior compartment of the thigh. It also produces one ventral division nerve, the **obturator nerve,** which supplies the medial compartment of the thigh. In the **sacral plexus,** several small branches supply

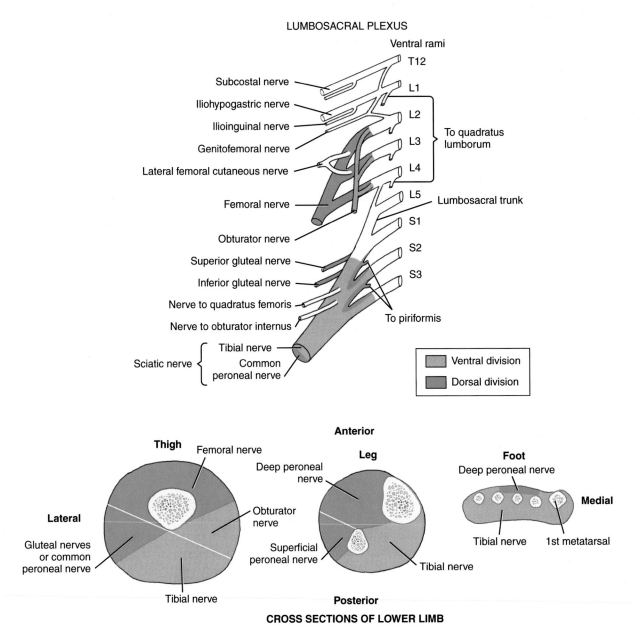

FIGURE 15-1
Organization and distribution of the lumbosacral plexus.

the muscles in the gluteal region. Muscles that arise from the ilium are developmentally dorsal; thus the **superior** and **inferior gluteal nerves** and the **nerve to the piriformis** supply them. Muscles that arise from the pubis or ischium are developmentally ventral; thus the **nerve to the quadratus femoris** and the **nerve to the obturator internus** supply them. The remaining nerve, the **sciatic nerve,** is a compound nerve containing the **common peroneal nerve** (dorsal division) and the **tibial nerve** (ventral division). The common peroneal nerve supplies the only muscle in the lateral compartment of the thigh (short head of the biceps femoris) then supplies the anterior and lateral compartments of the leg and the dorsal compartment of the foot. The tibial nerve supplies the posterior compartment of the thigh and leg and the plantar compartment of the foot.

Dissection

Examine the posterior abdominal body wall. **Identify** the **medial** and **lateral arcuate ligaments** and the **psoas major** and the **quadratus lumborum muscles** that emerge respectively from under the ligaments (**N263; G2.72; GY173; C252**). The psoas major combines with the **iliacus** to form the **iliopsoas,** sharing a common tendon of insertion on the **lesser trochanter** of the femur.

Clean away the **parietal peritoneum** and any **extraperitoneal fat** so as to expose the nerves of the posterior abdominal wall (**N267; G2.72; GY186; C253, 256**).

Identify the following nerves:
Subcostal
Iliohypogastric
Ilioinguinal
Lateral cutaneous nerve of the thigh
Femoral
Genitofemoral
Obturator
Lumbosacral trunk
Sacral plexus

Note the point of first appearance of each nerve and its relationship to surrounding structures. This process will help you to confirm your identifications. The **subcostal nerve** (T12) emerges from under the lateral arcuate ligament, following the twelfth rib until it penetrates the transversus abdominis. The **iliohypogastric nerve** (L1) and

the **ilioinguinal nerve** (L1) emerge from under the medial arcuate ligament deep to the psoas major. These nerves cross the **quadratus lumborum,** after which the iliohypogastric penetrates the transversus abdominis, and the ilioinguinal continues along the crest of the ilium.

TIP The pattern of the iliohypogastric and ilioinguinal nerves is often variable. They may emerge from the medial arcuate ligament either separately or remain united for some distance.

The **genitofemoral nerve** (L1-L2) penetrates the psoas muscle, emerging from its anterior surface and continuing along its length. The **lateral femoral cutaneous nerve** (L2-L3) appears lateral to the psoas and courses across the iliacus. The **femoral nerve** (L2-L4) is found further inferiorly on the lateral side of the psoas where it joins the **external iliac artery** and vein on their way through the femoral ring.

Pull the psoas laterally, and, on its medial side, **locate** the **obturator nerve** (L2-L4), which passes through the obturator membrane foramen. Just medial to the obturator is the **lumbosacral trunk** (L4-L5). This nerve bridges the lumbar and sacral plexuses and forms the most cranial roots of the sciatic nerve. The remaining roots of the sacral plexus are difficult to see within the true pelvis.

The psoas major has very little connective tissue within its belly (in beef, this cut of meat is the tenderloin, or filet mignon). Therefore it can be removed piecemeal by blunt dissection to expose the roots of the lumbar plexus.

Remove the psoas major on the right side of the cadaver, sparing specific nerves that penetrate the muscle.
Review the vasculature remaining in the **retroperitoneal space** (**N264, 265; G2.63; GY182, 183; C253**).
Trace the bifurcation of the abdominal aorta into the common iliac arteries, followed by the subsequent bifurcation into internal and external iliac arteries. **Note** also the parallel course of the common iliac veins and their tributaries.
Cut the inferior vena cava and abdominal aorta below the renal vessels, and **reflect** them inferiorly.
Inspect the lumbar vertebrae and sacrum. **Notice** the angle (**lumbosacral angle**) between the lumbar spine and the sacrum marking the **sacral promontory.**

Examine the **anterior longitudinal ligament** of the vertebral column. The superficial fibers are long and span several intervertebral joints. The deep fibers are short, spanning adjacent vertebrae, and they intermingle with the fibers of the **intervertebral discs.**

Using a bone saw, **remove** a quarter section of several vertebral bodies and intervertebral discs by making a sagittal section at the midline and a connecting frontal section.

Examine the structure of the cancellous bone within the vertebral bodies. **Turn** to the intervertebral disc. **Note** its laminar structure (Figure 15-2). *Can you differentiate between the **annulus fibrosus** and the **nucleus pulposus**? What changes occur in the intervertebral disc with age?*

The intervertebral disc is fibrocartilage, as also found in the symphysis pubis and some articular cartilages. Bundles of collagen fibers lie within the ground substance of hyaline cartilage matrix. Sparse chondrocytes lie scattered among the collagen fibers. Within alternating laminae, the bundles are oriented in regular spiral fashion. The nucleus pulposus binds water, rendering it uncompressible. It bulges outward when weight is applied to the vertebral column. The annulus resists tension because of this bulging.

With the psoas completely removed, you may be able to locate the stout **iliolumbar ligaments** spanning between the transverse processes of L4 and L5 and the ilium (**N353; G3.7; GY204; C253**).

Carefully pull the nerves to one side, and **clean away** obscuring muscle and fascia. The iliolumbar ligaments are very strong and play a significant role in preventing anterior slippage of the L5 vertebra on the sacrum (i.e., spondylolisthesis).

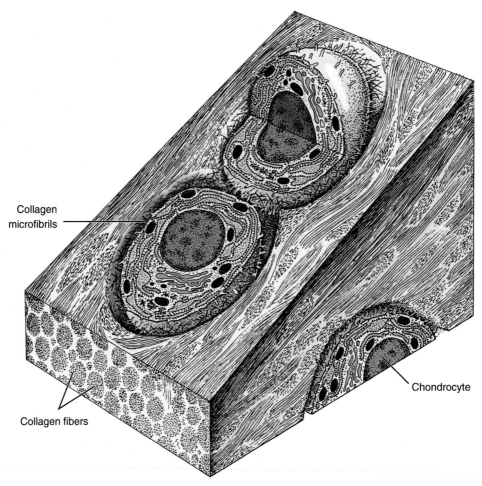

Collagen microfibrils

Collagen fibers

Chondrocyte

FIGURE 15-2

Histoarchitecture of the intervertebral disc showing arrangement of collagen fibers supported by chondrocytes. *(Modified from Krstic RV: General histology of the mammal, Berlin, 1984, Springer-Verlag.)*

Exercises

1. Color in and label on the figure below the branches of the lumbosacral plexus.

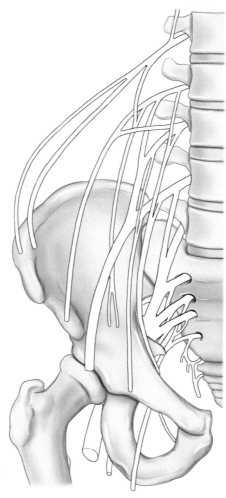

2. Draw in the iliolumbar ligaments on the figure below. How do they resist shear at the lumbosacral joint? Indicate with arrows the torques about the joint.

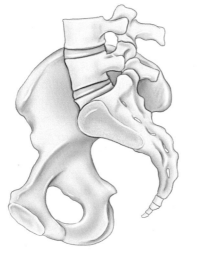
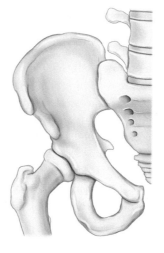

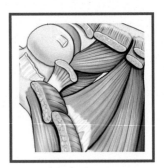

Anterior and Medial Thigh

LAB OBJECTIVES

In this exploration the anterior and medial compartments of the thigh will be examined, and the anatomy of the hip joint will be exposed. After completing this dissection the student should be able to:

- Describe the cutaneous innervation and distribution of dermatomes in this region.
- Describe the attachments, innervations, and actions of the quadriceps, adductors, and other muscles of the anterior and medial compartment.
- Define the femoral triangle and its contents.
- Discuss the bony and ligamentous anatomy of the pelvis and the hip joint.

CASE STUDY

Hip and Knee Pain

Mario is a 66 **y/o** retired chef who is being seen by a local orthopedic surgeon for an evaluation of his **L** hip and knee pain (4/10) that is aggravated when he ties his shoes every morning. The patient states that the pain decreases during the day, but, by bedtime, he really needs to lie down. He indicates that the pain is worse in the knee when he is standing or just moving around. Mario is an active man who retired from 20 years of long hours of standing while cooking as the head chef at a gourmet establishment. He currently takes daily walks and rides a bicycle on occasion to pain tolerance. He lives alone. His **PHM** includes **MI, CHF,** and **HTN,** all of which are currently managed with beta-blockers, diuretics, and anticoagulant medications. The physician's evaluation suggests normal **AROM** and **PROM** in **B** knees and ankles, **B left extremity DTRs are 2, – clonus, B left extremity** normal sensation, **AROM** or **PROM** of the **R** hip is

decreased with slight hip flexion contracture and pain on **contractile muscle testing (CMT)**. Posture is slightly kyphotic. During the evaluation, the physician asks him to demonstrate walking with a cane in his left hand, and the pain decreases immediately. Radiographic study reveals markedly decrease **R** hip joint space with a corrosive appearance of the femoral head.

Identification of the Anatomy

The hip anatomy must be clearly understood because, clinically, patients with hip conditions are commonly seen in hospitals and clinics. The hip joint complex is a very mobile and stable region surrounded by large musculature and a strong capsule to maintain body weight, balance, and negotiate triplanar motion in multiaxial functions. Particular attention needs to be focused on the anterior and posterior dissections because these areas are compromised during various surgical procedures. Note especially the various neurovascular structures during dissection.

Appreciate the following structures during dissection:

Musculature:
 The hip region
 Superficial:
  Gluteal group
  Quadriceps group
  Sartorius
  Adductor group
  Hamstring group
  Obturator exteruns
  Gemelli
  Tensor fascia latae
  Iliacus
  Psoas
  Piriformis
Joint complex:
 Capsule
 Head of the femur
 Acetabulum
 Greater and lesser trochanters
 ASIS
 AIIS
 PSIS
 PIIS
 Sacroiliac joint
Ligaments:
 Iliofemoral
 Ischiofemoral
 Pubofemoral
 Sacrotuberous
 Inguinal
 Interosseous
Soft-tissue, vascular, and nerve components:
 Femoral triangle (nerve, artery, and vein)
 Medial and lateral circumflex artery
 Deep femoral artery

Questions

1. Given the patient's history, signs and symptoms, and results of the evaluation, what can you suggest that makes this patient's pain worse?
2. Do you think this condition is a *degenerative* or an *acute* condition?

Discussion

Patients who have knee or hip pain need to be thoroughly evaluated as to the primary diagnosis. In many cases, a patient who complains of knee pain is really having issues with the hip on the ipsilateral side because hip pain neurologically *refers* to the knee.

Such is the case with this patient. He has **osteoarthritis** of the hip joint, not **rheumatoid arthritis**, which is a very different disease. His signs and symptoms are classic in that he has early morning pain and stiffness, he feels better in ambulation when he uses a cane because it reduces joint reaction forces, his films reveal joint space loss, and his work history suggests a profession that constantly bears weight on the joint. The condition of osteoarthritis can be managed by medications. However, when the pain becomes intolerable, most of these patients tend to undergo a surgical procedure called a total hip arthroplasty **(THA)** to replace the diseased joint components.

Preparation

Refer to the articulated skeleton (N486-489; G5.22; GY273; C265, 266, 430, 431), and identify the following landmarks of the pelvis and proximal femur:

 Symphysis pubis
 Pectin pubis
 Obturator foramen
 Superior and inferior rami of the pubis
 Greater and lesser trochanters of the femur
 Trochanteric fossa
 Intertrochanteric line and crest
 Pectineal line
 Medial and lateral lips of the linea aspera

Review the cutaneous innervation to the anterior and medial thigh (N538, 539, 544; G5.5; GY346, 347; C364, 367, 368) and the distribution of the dermatomes (N543; G5.7; GY346, 347; C364). The cutaneous nerves will be reflected in the skin flaps. The extremities have two sets of veins. The deep veins travel with the arteries and bear their names. In addition, a superficial set of veins can be found that travel largely in the superficial fascia. In the lower extremity, the largest of these veins is the **great saphenous vein**, which approximates the pre-axial border of the limb. Locate its position on the cadaver (N544; G5.10; GY344; C368). Take care to preserve and leave it intact when reflecting the skin.

Dissection

Remove the skin and superficial fascia from the anterior and medial thigh to just below the knee. Leave the great saphenous vein in place. **Notice** that the great saphenous vein penetrates the deep fascia through the **fossa ovalis** to reach the **femoral vein.** The deep fascia is very thick and is called the **fascia latae.**

Review the contents of the femoral triangle (**N500; G5.17, 5.18; GY290; C377**), and **trace** the course of the **femoral nerve** (L2-L4) to the muscles of the anterior compartment (**N501, 538; G5.23; GY291; C364, 379**).

Identify each muscle: **pectineus, iliopsoas, sartorius, rectus femoris, vastus lateralis, medialis,** and **intermedius,** and determine their attachments and actions (**N490, 491; G5.22; GY288, 289; C371, 430**).

TIP The contents of the femoral triangle (and other sites of major neurovascular bundles located in the popliteal fossae, axillae, and cubital fossae) can be remembered by reference to the acronym NAVEL: **N**erve, **A**rtery, **V**ein, **E**mpty space, **L**ymphatics.

Cut the pectineus muscle parallel to the inguinal ligament, and **reflect** it (occasionally, pectineus muscle has a dual innervation, receiving a branch from the obturator nerve).

The muscles of the medial compartment of the thigh are innervated by the **obturator nerve** (L2-L4). It emerges from the pelvis through the obturator foramen (**N501, 539; G5.23, 5.29; GY291; C364, 379**). The muscles of this compartment are largely adductors of the hip.

Identify the **gracilis** and the **adductor longus** muscles.

Section the adductor longus, and **reflect** it to reveal the **adductor brevis** (**N492, 493; G5.20; GY286, 288, 289; C374, 375, 378**).

Section the adductor brevis to expose fully the **adductor magnus.** This muscle has two parts and two innervations. The obturator nerve innervates the more proximal pubofemoral part. The ischiocondylar part, also called the *hamstrings part,* is innervated by the tibial portion of the sciatic nerve (L4). Between these two parts is an opening, a ligamentous **adductor hiatus.**

Identify the **obturator externus.** Unlike the other muscles of the medial compartment, the obturator externus is a lateral rotator of the hip.

Trace the femoral artery, and **identify** the **deep femoral artery** (**N500, 501; G5.8, 5.18; GY592; C364, 377,**

379). Its perforating branches supply the posterior compartment.

The femoral artery, vein, and **saphenous nerve** (a branch of the femoral nerve) continue within a connective tissue sheath called the **adductor canal.** The **artery** and **vein** pass through the adductor hiatus to reach the popliteal fossa, but the saphenous nerve becomes superficial and passes inferomedial to the knee.

EXPOSURE OF THE HIP JOINT (FIGURE 16-1)

Palpate the **anterior superior iliac spine** on the cadaver. With reference to this prominent landmark, **locate** the hip on an articulated skeleton. It lies just inferior to the midpoint of the inguinal ligament.

Section the neurovascular bundle within the femoral triangle.

Cut the sartorius a few centimeters from its origin. Then **cut** the iliopsoas and the pectineus parallel to the inguinal ligament, and **reflect** them.

Locate the obturator externus and section it (**N501; G5.29; GY291; C378**). **Section** the remaining muscles of the medial compartment at staggered levels so their ends can be more readily realigned. While an assistant extends and externally rotates the thigh, **incise** the anterior joint capsule obliquely, permitting the head of the femur to dislocate anteriorly.

TIP Place a block under the pelvis to achieve a greater range of extension at the hip.

The capsule is reinforced anteriorly by the **iliofemoral ligament (Y-ligament of Bigelow).**

Cut the **ligamentum teres** (**N487; G5.29-5.33; GY278, 279; C433**). You might consider sectioning the femoral neck within the capsule and removing the **head** altogether. This action will permit a better view of both the head and the **acetabulum.**

Examine the condition of the articular cartilage on the femoral head. *Do you see any erosions of the hyaline cartilage?* **Examine** the **lunate articular surface** of the acetabulum. Its margin is extended by the fibrocartilaginous **labrum.** The inferior horns of the lunate surface are bridged by the **transverse acetabular ligament** (**N487; G5.30; GY277; C433**), which permits the neurovascular supply to reach the head of the femur by passing below it.

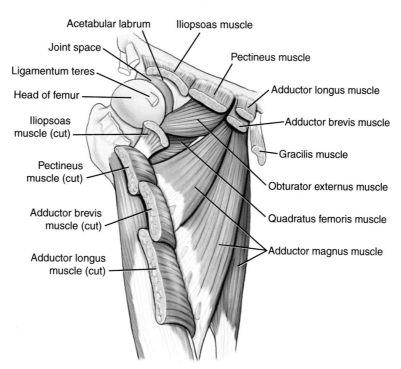

FIGURE 16-1
Exposure of the hip joint.

Exercises

1. Explain how the obturator externus can be a lateral rotator of the hip. Indicate by drawing free hand a superior view of the joint, indicating the axis of rotation of the joint and the line of pull of the muscle.

2. What do sportscasters mean when they refer to a *pulled groin* or groin injury? What is the anatomic basis for this expression?

3. Consider the compartmentalization of the thigh in cross-section. Label the compartments and indicate the nerves associated with each compartment and whether they are dorsal or ventral division on the figure below.

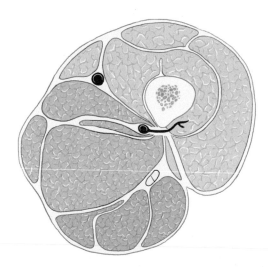

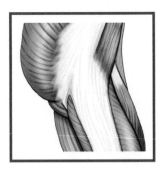

Gluteal Region and Posterior and Lateral Thigh

LAB OBJECTIVES

In this exploration, we examine two groups of muscles that are important in maintaining bipedal posture. They are particularly significant in the early period of the stance phase after heel strike. On completion of this lab the student should be able to:

- Describe the bony and ligamentous anatomy of the posterior pelvis and sacrum.
- Identify the attachments, innervation, and function of the gluteals and hamstrings.
- Describe the external rotators of the hip and their role in gait.
- Determine the course and distribution of the sciatic nerve.
- Describe the function of the fascia latae and the iliotibial band.

CASE STUDY

Patrolling the Highways

Lamont is a 40 **y/o** member of the Idaho State Highway Patrol and spends 10 hours a day keeping the freeways safe and traffic moving. He comes to a rural health clinic with **R** buttock pain of 1-month duration, which seems to refer to the lateral thigh and posterior leg. Lamont suggests that the pain occurs when he spends time in his newly issued patrol car. He also notices that the pain is worse when he wears his duty belt. He states that the belt is rather bulky and weighs approximately 10 kg, with more of the weight distributed on the right side owing to the placement of his firearm, ammunition, handcuffs, and other equipment. He is required to wear the belt on duty. The pain subsides after his shift but lingers for several hours. His **PMH** and systems review are unremarkable.

He denies any specific trauma or back pain over the years and is concerned that the pain may get worse and may interfere with his job duties.

Identification of the Anatomy

Isolate the bony anatomy, muscles, and specific nerves of the gluteal region.

Appreciate the following structures during dissection:

PSIS
PIIS
Greater and lesser sciatic notches
Greater and lesser trochanters of the femur
Lateral border of the sacrum
Sacroiliac joint
Ischial tuberosity
Gluteus maximus and medius and minimus muscles

Internal and external rotator muscles of the hip
Sciatic nerve

Questions

1. What may be the possible relationship among the new patrol car, the duty belt, and the pain Lamont is experiencing?
2. What are the anatomic structures compromised in the sitting position with the belt on?
3. Why would the pain *refer* into the buttock and lateral side of the thigh?
4. How can you differentiate between the pain from muscle or nerve?

Discussion

Though the gluteal muscles are generally large, they are not immune to external forces even if the forces are minimal. In the case of Lamont, minimal but constant pressure of the duty belt and the new seat in his patrol car may be the issues causing the pain. Wallets that are too thick and apply pressure over the buttocks can also cause this type of pain. This case revealed compression directly over the sciatic nerve **(nerve compression syndrome)** and the piriformis muscle, leading to pain and muscular spasm. This constant pressure may ignite muscle spasm and referred pain. Some patients also have **Piriformis Syndrome** in which the actual muscle is tight, which can cause similar symptoms. In rare instances (<2%), the sciatic nerve pierces the piriformis, which can cause constant discomfort. Patients in Lamont's situation can be treated through ergonomic alterations, stretching, and strengthening of the structures that may be compromised. Therapists should take the time to obtain a thorough history, conduct an evaluation and examination, and possibly perform a work-site evaluation to get a clear picture of the patient's problem. In this case, the problem was addressed by making a slight modification of the patrol car seat and shifting some of the accessories on the duty belt to the opposite side.

Preparation

On the articulated skeleton, identify on the **pelvis** (N486, 253; G5.31, 3.3; GY274, 275; C265, 266, 273):
  Posterior superior iliac spine
  Posterior inferior iliac spine
  Greater sciatic notch
  Ischial spine
  Lesser sciatic notch
  Ischial tuberosity
  Anterior, posterior, and inferior gluteal lines
  Iliac tubercle
Identify on the **femur** (N489; G5.22; GY276, 284; C430, 431):
  Trochanteric fossa
  Greater trochanter
  Intertrochanteric crest
  Lesser trochanter
  Gluteal tuberosity
Identify on the **tibia** (N495, 496; G5.22; GY284; C446, 447):
  Gerdy's tubercle
  Facet for the head of the fibula
  Medial and lateral tibial condyles
  Groove for the insertion of the semimembranosus

Dissection

Place the cadaver in a prone position, and **remove** the remaining skin from the gluteal region and posterior and lateral thigh.

Clean the surface of the **gluteus maximus** muscle (N495; G5.25; GY281; C390, 391).

Define its superior margin, and **differentiate** it from the **gluteal aponeurosis** over the **gluteus medius**.

Note the different fiber direction of the two muscles. With blunt dissection, **pass** first your fingers and then a probe deep to the belly of the gluteus maximus as far medially as possible, near its attachment to the sacrum.

Cut to the probe, sectioning the muscle and reflecting it laterally.

> **TIP** Note that some fibers of the gluteus maximus arise from the sacrotuberous ligament. Use a scalpel to detach these fibers close to their attachment to the ligament.

Locate the branches of the **inferior gluteal nerve** (L5-S2). It emerges from the **greater sciatic foramen** inferior to the **piriformis** muscle to supply the gluteus maximus (N502, 503; G5:26, 5.27; GY282, 283; C393).

The fibers of **gluteus medius** and **gluteus minimus** are parallel, and the muscles overlap, similar to roof shingles. Frequently, the intervening fascia is obliterated, and the two bellies cannot be easily separated. The plane of separation should be indicated by the **superior gluteal** nerve (L5-S1), which travels between them and gives off branches to each. The nerve first emerges from the **greater sciatic foramen** superior to the **piriformis**. The piriformis is often called the *key* to the gluteal region, and the greater sciatic notch is the *keyhole*. Inferior to the piriformis, the **sciatic nerve** emerges as well (although it may be split, with portions penetrating the piriformis or emerging superior to it; e.g., **G5.28**).

In addition to the piriformis are five additional lateral rotators. The lateral rotators can be remembered by the phrase, *"Please, GO! GO Quickly!"* referring, in order, to the **piriformis, superior gemellus, obturator internus, inferior gemellus, obturator externus,** and **quadratus femoris (N503; G5.27; GY281; C387).**

TIP Note that the obturator internus muscle is mostly tendinous once it crosses the lesser sciatic notch and may be fused to the bellies of the gemelli. The tendon of the obturator externus is considerably deeper and is found by separating the bellies of the inferior gemellus and the quadratus femoris.

Find the **nerve to the obturator internus** (L5-S1), which also supplies the superior gemellus, as well as the **nerve the quadratus femoris** (L5-S1), which supplies the inferior gemellus and passes deep to these muscles.

Find the stout **sacrotuberous ligament** that spans between the sacrum and the **ischial tuberosity** (N352, 353; G3.7; GY205; C430, 431). A second deeper ligament spans between the sacrum and **ischial spine—the sacrospinous ligament.** These two ligaments close off and divide the greater and lesser sciatic notches to form the **greater** and **lesser sciatic foramina.**

Consider the lateral thigh. Note the thickening of the **fascia latae** extending from the **tubercle of the iliac crest** to **Gerdy's tubercle** on the **lateral tibial condyle.** This thickening is the **iliotibial (IT) band.** Inserting on the IT band posteriorly are fibers of the gluteus maximus, whereas, anteriorly, inserts the **tensor fascia latae** muscle. The latter muscle is innervated by the **superior gluteal nerve** (L4-L5).

Clean away the remaining deep fascia, leaving the IT band in place.

The muscles of the posterior compartment of the thigh are collectively known as the **hamstrings.** These muscles include the **semitendinosus,**

Clinical Note

Iliotibial band friction syndrome (ITBFS)

The most common cause of lateral knee pain in runners is ITBS, although it can occur in any athlete who experiences repetitive knee flexion. As the knee approaches 30 degrees of flexion, at and shortly after foot strike, the posterior portion of the IT band rubs over the lateral epicondyle. The resulting friction may produce inflammation, hyperplasia, fibrosis, and mucoid degeneration in the soft tissue of the lateral synovial recess. As inflammation progresses, the impingement zone increases, thereby decreasing the range of pain-free motion. When the knee is completely extended, the IT band lies anterior to the lateral epicondyle. When it is deeply flexed, it lies posterior to it (Figure 17-1). When walking or running downhill, the angle of the knee at foot strike is reduced, and the IT band remains in the impingement zone longer. Some lower limb abnormalities may predispose individuals to ITBS, such as leg-length disparities, excessive Q-angle (i.e., the angle formed by a line drawn from the anterior-superior iliac spine to central patella and a second line drawn from central patella to tibial tubercle), and excessive foot **varus.** On clinical examination, the patient may have a positive Ober and Noble tests which indicate a tight IT.

semimembranosus, and the **biceps femoris (N495; G5.25; GY287; C390, 391).** The biceps femoris has two heads. The short head arises from the shaft of the femur and inserts on the lateral side of the head of the fibula. It receives its innervation from a branch of the **fibular portion of the sciatic nerve** (L5-S1). The short head is sometimes called the *lateral compartment of the thigh.* In contrast, the long head of the biceps femoris along with the remaining hamstrings receive their innervation from the **tibial component of the sciatic nerve** (L5-S2). The tendon of the **semitendinosus** joins those of the **gracilis** and **sartorius** to form the **pes anserinus,** or *goosefoot,* which inserts on the **medial tibial condyle.** Determine the remaining attachments of the hamstrings, and assess their actions.

The **adductor magnus** forms the floor of the posterior compartment.

Note the perforating braches from the **deep femoral artery** penetrating the muscle. **Locate** the **popliteal artery and vein** where they emerge from the **adductor hiatus.**

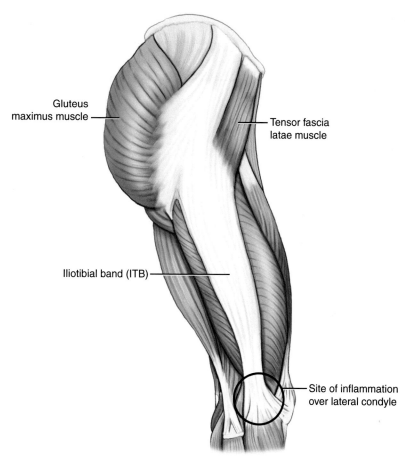

FIGURE 17-1

Lateral aspect of the thigh and hip indicating muscles. Site of pain in Iliotibial Band Friction Syndrome (ITBFS).

Exercises

1. Consider the angle of the femur to the perpendicular (valgus angle). In light of this arrangement, what might be the function of the IT band?

2. The gluteus medius is described as an abductor of the thigh. What function does it serve when the foot is planted?

3. Draw on the figure below the attachments of the muscles of the gluteal region.

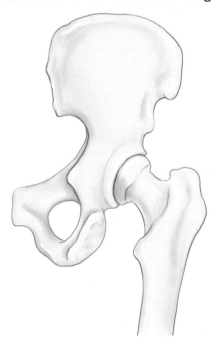

4. Draw in the sacrotuberous and sacrospinous ligaments on the figure below. Indicate the estimated line of the center of gravity of the body. Potential to resist non-axial movement at the sacroiliac joint ligaments.

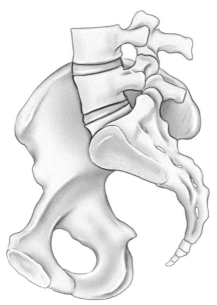

5. The piriformis is known as the *key* to the gluteal region. Draw in and list the neurovascular structures lying above (suprapiriformic) and below (infrapiriformic) the muscle on the figure below.

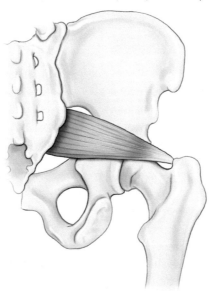

LAB EXPLORATION **18**

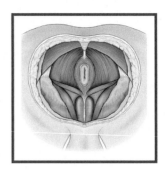

Perineum and Ischiorectal Fossa

LAB OBJECTIVES

In this lab the structures that comprise the pelvic floor are examined. On completion of this lab the student should be able to:

- Identify the neurovascular supply to the perineal region.
- Identify the muscles of the pelvic floor.
- Describe the relationship of the structures of the urogenital and anal triangles that perforate the pelvic floor.

CASE STUDY

Loss of Intimacy

Candice is a 35 **y/o** mother of four who **c/o** distal sacral pain **(coccydynia)** and buttock pain that has come and gone for the last 2 months after taking a fall while snowboarding. Candice gave birth to her daughter 1 year ago and had a difficult delivery. She indicates that physical position changes do not seem to minimize symptoms. She also has difficulty with **B/B** functions, claiming that they are painful. She relates a big problem of consistent diffuse pelvic pain during and after sexual intercourse **(dyspareunia).** She suggests that her current exercise regime has been less than optimal because she experiences pain in her legs even after trying short bouts of exercise. Her **PMH** includes a hernia repair 3 years ago. She also underwent varicose vein removal.

Identification of the Anatomy

Review the anatomy in Lab Exploration 8. Identify the bony landmarks, muscles, nerves, and other structures.

Appreciate the following structures during dissection:

Ischial tuberosity and spine

Symphysis pubis
Coccyx
Sacrotuberous ligament
Gluteus maximus
Levator ani muscle
Coccygeus muscle
Deep transverse perineal muscle
External and internal sphincter

Questions

1. Can you postulate which of her symptoms are musculoskeletal in nature? Vascular?
2. From this patient's history, can you suggest any *risk factors* that may suggest *red flags* for a more serious condition?

Discussion

This clinical presentation is not uncommon for patients with a laundry list of possible diagnoses. Pelvic and sacral pain can mask serious disease process in almost every system of the body. The symptom of distal sacral pain may be a fractured coccyx, and the pelvic pain during intercourse may directly relate to muscle spasm or tightness in the focal musculature of the pelvic diaphragm or **pelvic floor tension**

139

myalgia. The pain during sexual intercourse may also be related to scar adhesions or possibly to positional alterations of the uterus, bladder, or vagina. Her leg pain during exercise **(claudication)** may be an indication of peripheral vascular disease **(PVD)**, which may lead to numerous serious vascular complications. The examiner must be precise in his or her evaluation to tease out information that would alert the examiner to a need for a medical referral. The **red flags** for possible pelvic cancer may include marked weight loss, vaginal bleeding, abdominal pain, and fatigue. Any one of these *flags* in this patient would warrant the need for an immediate medical referral.

Preparation

Review the bony boundaries of the pelvic outlet:
Symphysis pubis
Inferior ramus of the pubis
Inferior ramus of the ischium
Ischial spine
Ischial tuberosity
Coccyx

Anatomic Overview

The perineal region is a diamond-shaped area defined by the coccyx, symphysis pubis, and ischial tuberosities (N357, 359; G3.52, 3.53, 3.55; GY 215, 244; C294, 318). A line joining the ischial tuberosities separates the **urogenital triangle** and the **anal triangle.** Skeletal muscles that support the pelvic viscera form the pelvic diaphragm. These muscles are collectively designated the **levator ani muscle.** It is composed of three parts: **puborectalis, pubococcygeus,** and **iliococcygeus** (N395; G3.62; GY245, 246; C21).

Dissection

Place the cadaver in prone position, and **locate** the **pudendal nerve** and the **internal pudendal artery** where they emerge from the infrapiriformic space

of the greater sciatic foramen (N411, 413; G3.60; GY253; C295, 319).
Trace their paths posterior to the sacrospinous ligament and anterior to the sacrotuberous ligament (Figure 18-1).

NERVES OF THE PERINEUM (N411, 413; G3.51, 3.60; GY253; C295, 319)

Incise the perimeter of the anus and, in the woman, the perimeter of the vulva as well. In the man, split the scrotum along the scrotal septum, separating the two halves laterally. **Make** an incision encircling the base of the penis.
Skin the anterior perineum to the margin of the inferior ramus of the pubis. The ischiorectal fossa is a fat-filled space located to either side of the anus.
Use scissor-technique to trace the pudendal nerve and internal pudendal artery, and **remove** the fat.
Expose the **external anal sphincter** and the levator ani muscle of the pelvic diaphragm.
Locate the **inferior rectal nerves and arteries,** branches of the **pudendal nerve,** and the **internal pudendal artery.** The lateral border of the ischiorectal fossa is formed by the obturator internus muscle. The **pudendal nerve** and the **internal pudendal artery** penetrate the fascia of the obturator internus muscle and pass through the **pudendal canal** (see Figure 18-1, *A*).

The perineal nerves and arteries, the second set of branches of the **pudendal nerve** and the **internal pudendal artery,** course toward the urogenital triangle. The superficial perineal pouch obscures the anterior portions of the levator ani. The **perineal membrane** bounds the superior pouch (Figure 18-2).

Locate and **clean** the **superficial transverse perineal muscle,** the **bulbospongiosus muscle,** and the **ischiocavernosus muscle** in both the male and the female pelvis.

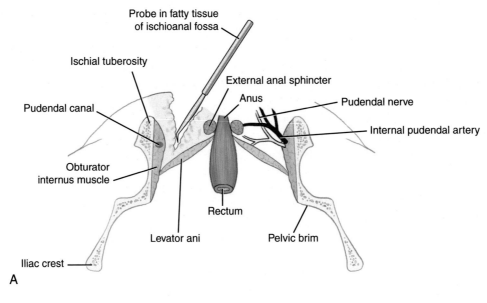

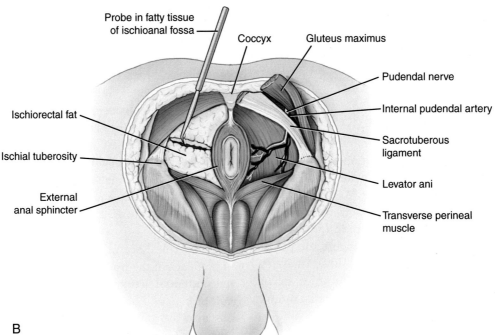

FIGURE 18-1
A, Coronal section through the ischiorectal fossa. **B,** Inferior view of the ischiorectal fascia.

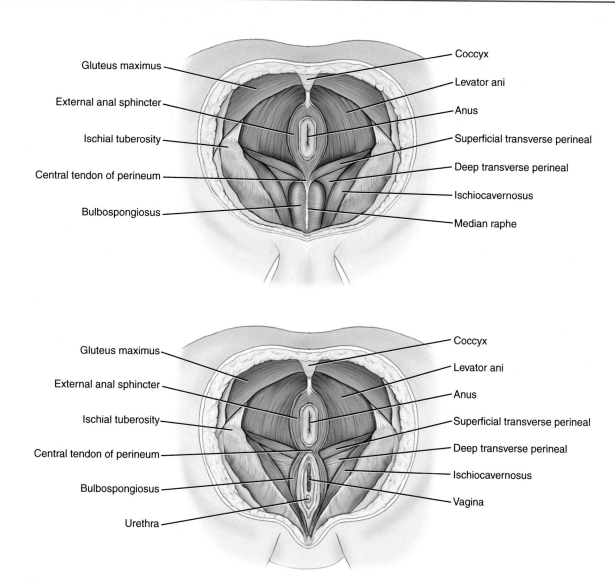

FIGURE 18-2
Inferior view of the male and female pelvic diaphragm.

Exercises

1. On the inferior view of the pelvis below, drawn in and label the muscles of the pelvic floor.

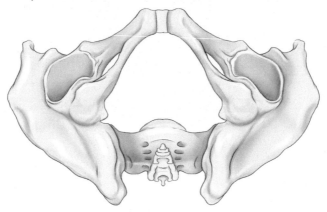

2. An exercise to strengthen the pelvic diaphragm is to voluntarily interrupt micturition (urination). What specific muscles are involved?

Popliteal Fossa and Knee Joint

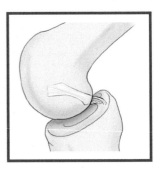

LAB OBJECTIVES

In this lab the visceral structures associated with the knee will be examined. The anatomy and function of the knee joint will be considered. On completion of this lab the student should be able to:

- Describe the bony landmarks of the distal femur, patella, proximal tibia, and fibula.
- Define the boundaries and contents of the popliteal fossa.
- Identify the pes anserinus (goosefoot).
- Describe the attachments and functions of the cruciate ligaments and menisci.

CASE STUDY

Post Partum Knee Pain

Greta is a 30 **y/o** woman who is being seen during a Saturday free clinic for the recreational athlete. She is being reviewed by a **PT** and an athletic trainer **(ATC)**. She is an avid runner and skier and is 2 months' postpartum with her second child. She was on bed rest on the recommendation of her physician for approximately 8 weeks because of **toxemia** (**HTN** during pregnancy) before delivery. She noticed **B** knee pain when she tried to regain her running regime to shed her pregnancy weight, and the pain was localized to her lateral knee margins. The pain is sometimes a 6/10 when she runs, but she indicates that it increases when going up and down stairs. She has stopped running but she would still like to lose the 30 lb she gained during pregnancy. Greta's physical examination appears normal, other than slight **crepitus** (grinding of the joint as it moves through a **ROM**) in **B** knees during full **ROM,** pain on manual muscle test **(MMT)** of the quadriceps, atrophy of **B VM** (i.e., vastus medialis), and a noticeable lateral facing of **B** patellae

and **pes planus** (flat feet). An additional clinical finding was a positive **apprehension sign** (i.e., pain and contraction when the patella is moved laterally on the **L**).

Identification of the Anatomy

The knee and thigh anatomy are intricately involved with the function of the lower extremity. The arthrologic feature of the knee is a composite of two articulations (femorotibial and patellofemoral), and they act in a uniaxial or biaxial motion, depending on position of the joint in flexion and extension. The knee joint presents a host of problems for individuals who are actively engaged in exercise activities, are overweight, or have a predisposition for arthritis. Pay close attention to the morphology of the femoral condyles, tibial plateau, patella, and the intra- and extracapsular structures.

Appreciate the following structures during dissection:

Musculature:
    Quadriceps group
    Hamstring group

Gracilis
Sartorius
Plantaris
Gastrocsoleus complex
Popliteus
Tibialis groups
Fibular group
Joint complex:
  Tibia femoral articulations
  Patellofemoral articulations
  Supra- and infrapatellar spaces
  Menisci
Ligaments:
  Tibial collateral ligament
  Fibular collateral ligament
  Anterior cruciate ligament
  Posterior cruciate ligament
  Ligament of Wrisberg
  Transverse ligament
  Coronary ligament
Soft tissue and neurovascular:
  Iliotibial band
  Pes anserinus
  Popliteal neurovascular bundle
  Overlying fascia of the proximal lower leg

Questions

1. Given the signs, history, and symptoms of this case, what would be the possible biomechanical cause leading to this pain?
2. Can you predict what alignment or structures may be the culprits for the basis of this pain?

Discussion

The normal dynamics of knee joint function are interwoven with patellar alignment during functional movement. A person's strength, specific joint morphology, and weight are all involved in normal function of the knee in the sagittal and transverse planes. This patient has all the classic signs of **patellofemoral tracking syndrome (PFTS). PFTS** is more common in woman than men, may involve weakness of the medial musculature of the thigh, is enhanced by foot pronation, and is not uncommon when people try to exercise after a long respite from regular activity (e.g., after bed rest). Similar signs and symptoms may also appear with a **plica** (abnormally large fold of synovial tissue). In extreme conditions, a surgeon may perform a lateral release to move the patella medially for better alignment during motion.

Preparation

Refer to the articulated skeleton, and note the relationship of the femur to the tibia and patella. Normally the long axis of the femur intersects that of the tibia at an angle of approximately 185 to 195 degrees—the valgus angle.

Identify on the **femur** (N489; G5.22; GY276, 284; C430, 431):
  Medial and lateral condyles
  Medial and lateral epicondyles
  Patellar surface
  Popliteal surface
Identify on the **patella:**
  Vertical ridge
  Inferior, middle, and superior facets
  Medial vertical facet (odd facet)
Identify on the **tibia** (N495, 496; G5.22; GY284; C3446, 447):
  Medial and lateral condyles
  Intercondylar tubercles
  Tibial tuberosity
  Gerdy's tubercle
Identify on the **fibula:**
  Head
  Neck

The knee complex is composed of two articulations within a single joint capsule. These joints are the tibiofemoral joint and patellofemoral joint. The knee joint is commonly known as a hinge joint. However, it is more a condylar joint in which flexion-extension are combined with gliding and rolling and limited axial rotation.

Dissection

Place the cadaver in prone position, and **identify** the **popliteal fossa**—a diamond-shaped intermuscular space bounded by the hamstrings and the gastrocnemius. The roof of this space is formed by the deep fascia, and the floor is formed by the popliteal surface of the femur, knee joint capsule, and popliteus muscle. Its contents are the **popliteal artery** and **vein, sciatic nerve** (L4-S3) dividing to become the **common fibular** and **tibial nerves, lateral** and **medial sural cutaneous nerves** (L5-S1), and the **small saphenous vein** (N516; G5.36, 5.37; GY308; C412, 413).

Demonstrate the continuity of the femoral artery with the popliteal artery at the adductor hiatus (N512; G5.8; GY294, 295; C363). **Note** that it passes under the soleus via a tendinous arch (N517; G5.38; GY322; C416).

The sciatic nerve divides into its two components, the tibial nerve (ventral division nerve to the posterior compartment of the leg) and the common peroneal nerve (dorsal division to the anterior and lateral compartments of the leg). The medial sural cutaneous nerve arises from the tibial nerve; the lateral sural cutaneous nerve arises from the common peroneal nerve.

Identify the innervation fields of these nerves (N540; G5.5; GY347; C365, 367). The **small saphenous vein** is a superficial vein draining the posterolateral aspects of the leg before penetrating the deep fascia to join the **popliteal vein** (N545; G5.10; GY344; C382, 412).

Place the foot on a block to reduce tension on the gastrocnemius.

Separate the heads of the gastrocnemius to expose the **plantaris** and the **popliteus muscles. Identify** their attachments.

The plantaris will be considered in more detail later. The popliteus has been attributed with multiple functions, including flexion of the knee, unlocking the knee at the beginning of flexion, medial rotation of the tibia on the femur, and lateral rotation of the femur on the fixed tibia. However, electromyographic studies suggest that the popliteus *functions* to resist the tendency for the femur to rotate medially relative to the tibia during contraction of the powerful medial rotators of the hip, especially during the later part of stance phase of gait.

Two ligaments reinforce the posterior surface of the joint capsule. The first ligament is the **oblique popliteal ligament** (N511; G5.45; GY300; C438), which is an expansion of the semimembranosus tendon. The second ligament, the **arcuate popliteal ligament,** runs distally from the lateral femoral epicondyle to the posterior surface of the joint capsule; it is inferior, but roughly parallel to, the oblique ligament. Two fibrous bands arch over the popliteus to anchor it to the head of the fibula.

Open the posterior joint capsule, and **expose** the **posterior cruciate ligament** (PCL) on one knee (Figure 19-1). Arising from the lateral meniscus is

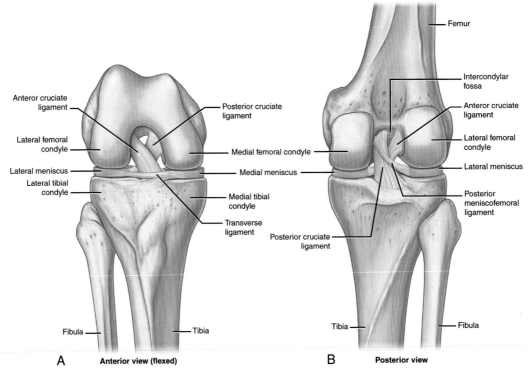

A   Anterior view (flexed)

B   Posterior view

FIGURE 19-1

The cruciate ligaments seen from **A,** anterior *(left)* and **B,** posterior *(right)* views. *(From Drake R et al: Gray's atlas of anatomy, Philadelphia, 2008, Churchil Livingstone.)*

the **posterior meniscofemoral ligament** (ligament of Wrisberg), which may be present and, if found, runs proximal to attach to the medial condyle of the femur posterior to the attachment of the PCL (N509; G5.12; GY302; C440).

Place the cadaver in a supine position. **Review** the attachments of the quadriceps femoris via the patella to the tibial tuberosity.

The most lateral fibers of the tendon of the vastus lateralis bypass the patella to insert on the front of the lateral tibial condyle as the **lateral patellar retinaculum** (N507; G5.40, 5.43, 5.44; GY300, 302; C435). Similarly, the most medial fibers of the tendon of the vastus medialis bypass the patella to insert on the front of the medial tibial condyle as the **medial patellar retinaculum.**

Review the insertions of the muscles of the thigh that act across the medial aspect of the knee joint.

Note the **pes anserinus** *(goosefoot)*—tendinous expansions of the **sartorius, gracilis,** and **semitendinosus** (recall the acronym SAGS). These three muscles represent three different compartments of the thigh and are innervated by three different nerves (N506; G5.21, 5.41; C414).

Identify the compartments and innervations of each. (If you have difficulty recalling which side of the knee the goosefoot is located, simply think of *M*other Goose and *m*edial.) The fourth muscle crossing the medial side of the knee is the **semimembranosus.**

Cut and **reflect** the tendons of the pes anserinus. Attempt to **locate** the **anserine bursa.** *Where else might you expect to find bursae about the knee?*

Clean and **expose** the **tibial collateral ligament** (N506; G5.46). It runs from the medial femoral epicondyle to the proximal tibial. Its fibers fuse to the joint capsule, and some fibers attach to the medial meniscus. *What movement does this ligament resist?*

Turn to the lateral aspect of the knee, and **review** the attachments of the iliotibial tract and the long and short head of the biceps femoris. (Associate *l*ong head of biceps femoris with *l*ateral.)

Cut and **reflect** the tendon of the biceps femoris to reveal the **fibular collateral ligament** (N506; G5.41; GY300; C440). It runs from the lateral femoral epicondyle to the head of the fibula and is separate from the joint capsule and the lateral meniscus. *What movement does this ligament resist?*

Make a transverse cut just above the patella, opening the joint capsule. **Explore** its extent. The expansive extension of the synovial cavity superior is the **suprapatellar bursa** (N507, 511; G5.47, 5.52; GY306; C441).

Flex the knee to expose the infrapatellar synovial fold (N507; G5.43; GY305; C436).

Clean away the synovium and fat to expose the **anterior** and **posterior cruciate ligaments** (N509; G5.44; GY302; C438). *How can the cruciate ligaments be intracapsular but extrasynovial* (N508; G5.52; GY303; C443)? The cruciate ligaments are named for their attachments to the tibia.

TIP Place your right foot directly in front of your left and your legs form the cruciate ligaments of your *right* knee. By rotating your hips, you will have a vivid representation of the impact of femoral rotation on the cruciate ligaments.

The posterior cruciate ligament is the stouter of the two ligaments. It resists anterior translation of the femur on the tibia (Figure 19-2). The anterior cruciate ligament is tension during extension of the knee, or when the femur is internally rotated on a fixed tibia. Not only is the anterior cruciate ligament stretched across the posterior cruciate ligament during that motion, but the narrow intercondylar cleft also has a scissoring effect. Such is even more the case in women, in whom the narrowness and depth of the fossae is often more pronounced.

Pull the tibia as far forward as possible, and **examine** the fibrocartilaginous menisci (N508; G5.46; GY303; C443). The **medial meniscus** is more C-shaped, whereas the **lateral meniscus** is more O-shaped.

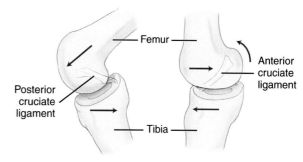

FIGURE 19-2

Functions of the cruciate ligaments of the knee seen in mediolateral view.

Clinical Note

Lachman's and anterior drawer test

The anterior cruciate ligament **(ACL)** is the weaker of the two ligaments and is taut in extension (G5.53). If it becomes torn, the tibial plateau can be pulled anteriorly forward more than 1 cm **(Anterior Drawer Test and the Lachman's Test)**. Sever the ACL, and examine the posterior cruciate ligament **(PCL)**. The PCL is stronger than the ACL and tightens on flexion and posterior displacement of tibia and is actually considered the *stabilizer* of the knee. If the PCL is torn, the tibia can be pushed posteriorly more than 1 cm—a positive **posterior drawer,** the **posterior lag** or drop sign tests. Young women have a higher incidence of ACL injuries than men secondary to a tighter femoral condylar notch, weak hamstrings, and possible hormonal changes.

TIP Think of the acronym **RSCO**—when looking down on your right-side tibia, the menisci approximate the letters **CO**.

Tears of the medial meniscus are 20 times more common than other tears because it is firmly attached to the tibial collateral ligament.

Observe the **transverse ligament** **(N509; G5.44; GY303; C443)**, which unites the anterior horns of the menisci.

Exercises

1. On the superior view of the tibia below, draw in the attachments of the ligaments spanning the knee joint.

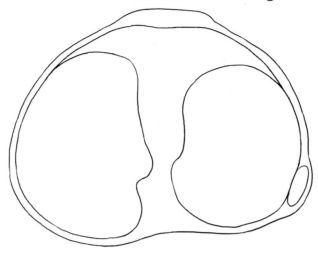

2. On the superior view of the tibia below, draw in the medial and lateral menisci and their attachments.

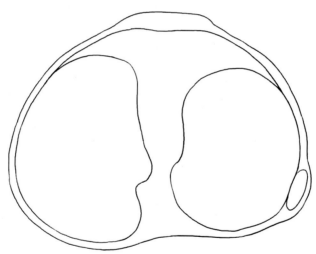

3. What structures restrict medial rotation of the femur relative to the tibia?

4. What structures restrict lateral rotation of the femur relative to the tibia? (Demonstrate with crossed legs.) The most frequent cause of isolated tears of anterior cruciate ligament is imposed lateral rotation of femur on the fixed tibia.

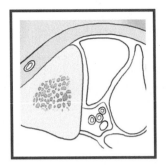

Leg and Dorsum of the Foot

> ### LAB OBJECTIVES
>
> In this lab the structures the crus, or leg, and dorsal compartment of the foot will be explored. On completion of this lab the student should be able to:
> - Describe the bony landmarks of the tibia and the fibula.
> - Identify superficial veins and cutaneous nerve fields.
> - Describe the deep fascia and the compartmental organization of the leg.
> - Identify muscle attachments, actions, and innervations.

CASE STUDY

Painful Mail Delivery

Fritz, a 46 **y/o** U.S. Postal Service letter carrier, was seen at a local physician's office immediately after he delivered the same physician's mail. Evidently, Fritz had just dropped off a package with the secretary, and as he was walking down the stairs outside the office, he lost his balance, and, in an effort to break his fall, he stepped forward with his **L** foot and felt significant pain and heard a *pop* in his leg. He was not able to stand on the **L** foot but managed to hobble up the stairs and alert the physician to the problem. The physician immediately examined him and found the following. The **R** left extremity **(LE)** was clear of disease and normal to examination. The **L LE** displayed edema below the knee, shortened gastrocsoleus complex, non–weight-bearing status, decreased **pedal pulses** (posterior tibial and dorsalis pedis arteries), exquisite point tenderness at the posterior aspect of the calcaneus, and a painful **+ Thompson's test** (manually squeezing of the belly of the gastrocnemius muscle with no passive dorsiflexion noted). The physician sent him to the **ER** for an x-ray examination and further orthopedic evaluation.

Identification of the Anatomy

The lower leg, ankle, and foot anatomy are vital to the understanding of functional weight-bearing activities and are considered some of the most abused areas of the human body, in light of the various tasks the structures are asked to perform. The anterior, posterior, and lateral compartments of the lower leg function to control distal triplanar foot movements, balance, and other proprioceptive tasks. This area contains several muscles that are biarticulate in nature and function to stabilize the many joints of the ankle and foot.

Appreciate the following structures during dissection:

Musculature:
   Gastrocsoleus grouping
   Fibularis group
   Extensor digitorum group
   Extensor hallucis group
   Flexor hallucis group
   Tibialis group
Joint complex:
   Talocrual
   Subtalar
   Midtarsal

Tarsal-metatarsal
Phalanges
Tibiofibular interosseous membrane
Ligaments:
    Anterior tibiofibular
    Anterior talofibular
    Tibiofibular group
    Fibular-calcaneal group
Soft tissue, vasculature and nerves:
    Flexor and extensor retinaculae, intramuscular
      fascia
    Neurovascular bundles (branches of the peroneal
      nerve, anterior-posterior tibial arteries)
    Fibular artery
    Dorsalis pedis artery
    Saphenous veins

Question

Given the immediate history and signs and symptoms of this patient, what would you surmise the problem to be with his lower leg, and what are the major structures involved?

Discussion

The compressive, tension, and shear forces produced by muscle contractions during general movement can be as high as 10 times the body weight in certain situations. The coupling of these forces with the various lever systems in the body can have devastating results on bone a soft tissue. Biologic tissues are generally viscoelastic and rate dependent, which suggests that they react very differently when loaded at various speeds. In this case, this patient actually avulsed a portion of the calcaneus through the tension created in the calcaneal (Achilles') tendon. Bone, when loaded slowly, is weak compared with tendon. The properties of soft tissues are important to remember during diagnosis, treatment, and rehabilitation of patients.

Preparation

Notice that the tibia is roughly triangular in cross-section at the mid shaft (N513, 514; G5.53, 5.59; GY309; C446, 447). It has **anterior, medial,** and **interosseus borders,** bounding **medial, lateral,** and **posterior surfaces.** The fibula has a somewhat twisted appearance, but it has **anterior** and **posterior borders** and a **medial crest.** An **interosseus border** courses adjacent to the anterior border. On the tibia, fibula and **interosseus membrane** identify the points of origin of the

leg muscles, and their tendon courses at the ankle, noting the associated bony landmarks (N515; G5.53, 5.59; GY319; C405, 420):

Oblique line
Soleal line
Medial malleolus
Lateral malleolus

Before reflecting the skin, review the tributaries of the **great saphenous vein** and the **lesser** or **small saphenous vein** (N544, 545; G5.10; GY344; C398, 412). These superficial veins lie with the superficial fascia and will likely be reflected with the skin flap. Next, review the distribution of the cutaneous nerve fields (N538, 540, 542; G5.5; GY546, 547; C366, 367). Identify the **medial cutaneous nerve** of the leg (continuation of the saphenous nerve [a branch of femoral nerve]), **medial and lateral sural cutaneous nerves** (sciatic nerve), and **superficial peroneal nerve** (L5-S2). *What dermatomes do these nerves involve* (N543; G5.7; GY346, 347; C364, 365)? Refer to the distribution of cutaneous innervation over the dorsum of the foot. Trace the **saphenous nerve, sural nerve,** and the **superficial peroneal nerve** into the foot. *What is the source of the sural nerve?* A small area of skin between the first and second digits is supplied by the **deep peroneal nerve** (L4-L5). The sole of the foot is supplied by branches of the tibial nerve, that is, the **medial calcaneal branches** and the **medial** and **lateral plantar nerves.**

Dissection

Place the cadaver in a supine position, and **reflect** the skin from the leg to just below the ankle.

Note the thickness of the deep fascia (crural fascia) over the anterior compartment. You will need to remove the fascia to expose and identify the muscles of the anterior compartment: **tibialis anterior** (L4-L5), **extensor digitorum longus** (L5-S1), **peroneus tertius** (L5-S1), and somewhat deeper the **extensor hallucis longus** (L5-S1) (N519; G5.53; GY324; C399).

Separate the tibialis anterior and the extensor digitorum longus to find the principal neurovascular bundle in the anterior compartment (N520; G5.54; GY325; C346). This bundle contains the **anterior tibial artery, tibial vein,** and the **deep peroneal**

Clinical Note

Anterior Tibial Compartment Syndrome

Patients suffering direct blunt soft tissue trauma, fracture, the application of tight casts, or even overuse, may compromise the lower leg, resulting in decreased blood perfusion and subsequent "compartment pressures." This, in turn may lead to decreased nerve function, atrophy of related musculature in the compartment, and possible necrosis of tissue. The anterior compartment of the lower leg is highly susceptible to this condition since it, as well as the lateral and posterior compartments, are confined by thick fascial and bony borders. In severe cases this is a limb threatening injury, which needs immediate operative decompression to resume normal blood flow. Absences of pulse, decreased sensation, pain on passive motion, and skin tightness are some of the classic signs and symptoms of this type of syndrome.

nerve. *What are the boundaries of the anterior compartment of the leg (N522; G5.91; GY328; C463)?*

Remove the skin from the dorsum of the foot. The skin is relatively thin on this surface. The deep fascia is reinforced in front of the ankle to prevent bowstringing of the extrinsic extensor tendons. These reinforced areas are called **retinaculae.**

Identify the **superior extensor retinaculum** and the Y-shaped **inferior extensor retinaculum (N530; G5.55; GY333; C407).** Note that the extrinsic extensor tendons are encompassed by **synovial sheaths.**

Trace the tendon of the **tibialis anterior** to its insertion on the medial cuneiform and base of the first metatarsal (N515; G5.53, 5.61; GY330; C405, 420).

Trace the tendons of the **extensor hallucis longus** and the **extensor digitorum longus.** The former inserts on the distal phalanx; the latter divides to form an extensor hood similar to that in the fingers. *Is a **peroneus tertius** present?* If so, **follow** its tendon to the base of the fifth metatarsal.

In contrast to the hand, the foot has a dorsal compartment occupied by intrinsic extensors of the digits.

Identify the **extensor hallucis brevis,** and **trace** its tendon to the distal phalanx of the hallux. Find the **extensor digitorum brevis,** and **trace** its

tendons to the extensor expansions of the second, third, and fourth toes. The muscles of the dorsal compartment are innervated by the **deep peroneal nerve.**

The anterior tibial artery continues into the dorsum of the foot as the **dorsalis pedis artery.** The pulse of the dorsalis pedis artery is readily palpable in most individuals. An important point to note is that, occasionally, the anterior tibial artery is a branch of the fibular artery.

Turn the cadaver into a prone position, and **completely remove** the skin from the leg. *Do not skin the sole of the foot at this time.*

Consider the lateral compartment, and **identify** the **peroneus longus** (L5-S2) and **peroneus brevis** (L5-S2) **(N521; G5.57; GY323; C404).** The tendons of the fibular muscles pass posterior to the lateral malleolus (Figure 20-1). They are held in place by the **superior** and **inferior fibular retinaculae.** The **superficial peroneal nerve** passes between the muscle bellies (N520; G5.54; GY326; C402).

TIP Note that the peroneus tertius, in spite of the similarity in names, is not part of the lateral compartment but is derived from the extensor digitorum longus and is part of the anterior compartment.

The **common peroneal nerve** runs subcutaneously across the fibular neck. At this point, it is susceptible to blunt trauma or compression. Damage to the nerve results in *foot drop*, wherein the patient cannot dorsiflex or evert the foot.

The posterior compartment of the leg is divided into superficial and deep regions. The superficial portion contains the **gastrocnemius** (S1-S2), the **soleus** (S1-S2), and the **plantaris** (S1-S2), which insert via a common **calcaneal (Achilles') tendon** on the calcaneus (N516, 517; G5.60; GY321; C413, 415, 416). This stout tendon is a significant elastic storage mechanism during running.

Cut the two heads of the gastrocnemius close to their origins on the femoral epicondyles, and **cut** the soleus along its origin at the soleal line of the tibia and the proximal fibula. **Reflect** them distally.

The deep portion of the posterior compartment contains the **tibialis posterior** (L4-L5), flanked by the **flexor digitorum longus** (S2-S3),

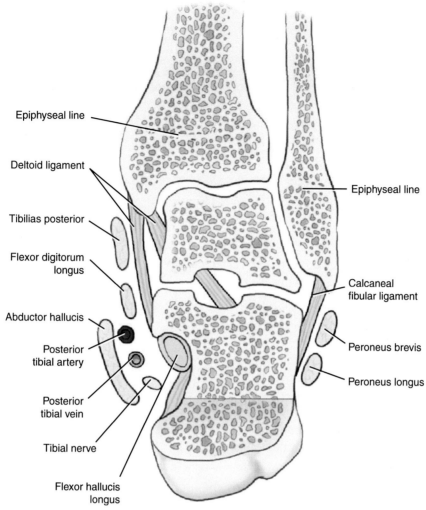

Epiphyseal line

Deltoid ligament

Tibilias posterior

Flexor digitorum longus

Abductor hallucis

Posterior tibial artery

Posterior tibial vein

Tibial nerve

Flexor hallucis longus

Epiphyseal line

Calcaneal fibular ligament

Peroneus brevis

Peroneus longus

FIGURE 20-1
Coronal section through the ankle.

and the **flexor hallucis longus** (S2-S3). The principle neurovascular bundle in the posterior compartment of the leg contains the **posterior tibial artery** and **vein** and the **tibial nerve** (N500; G5.73; C417, 419). The posterior tibial artery gives off the **fibular artery,** which remains in the posterior compartment but supplies the peroneal (fibular) muscles by way of branches perforating the intermuscular septum.

Posterior to the medial malleolus are the flexor tendons and neurovascular bundle (see Figure 20-1).

These structures are retained by the **flexor retinaculum.** A phrase might help you remember the sequence of structures moving from medial to lateral: *Tom, Dick, and very nervous Harry.*

Tom	**T**ibialis posterior tendon
Dick	Flexor **d**igitorum longus
And	Posterior tibial **a**rtery
Very	Posterior tibial **v**ein
Nervous	Tibial **n**erve
Harry	Flexor **h**allucis longus

Exercises

1. A herniation of the L5-S1 intervertebral disc compresses the S1 nerve root. In the figure below, draw in the region of radicular pain or sensory deficit resulting from compression of this S1 nerve root.

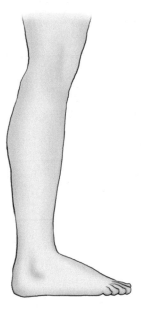

2. In the figure below, color in and label the structures seen in cross-section of the leg. Trace the boundaries of the anterior compartment.

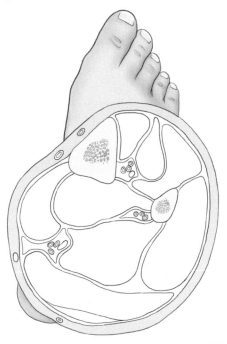

3. Given its superficial location at the fibular neck, the common peroneal nerve is the most commonly injured nerve in the leg. What motor deficits would be presented and how would they affect gait?

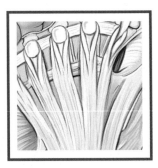

Plantar Foot and Ankle

LAB OBJECTIVES

In this lab, you will be exploring the layered anatomy of the plantar foot and ankle joint. After completing this lab, you should be able to:

- Describe the bony landmarks of the distal tibiofibula, tarsus, metatarsus, and phalanges.
- Identify the ligaments and movements of the distal tibiofibular, talocrural, subtalar, and remaining joints.
- Discuss the disposition and function of the transverse and longitudinal arches and supporting ligaments.
- Outline the layered organization of the foot musculature.

CASE STUDY

Painful First Steps

Jerome is a 65 **y/o** retired professor and has been a tennis player all his life. Recently, he has been training for a marathon with his son, who is an avid runner, and has set up a progressive training schedule with several other younger runners. He visits the local sports medicine clinic on Wednesday after a longer-than-expected run on Sunday. He sheepishly admits that he was trying to keep up the pace with the younger fellows, stating that he "overdid" the workout. His complaint today is that of pain on the plantar surface of the **R** foot, and it hurts most when he takes the first step after getting out of bed, but then the pain improves as the day goes on. He suggests that it may be a bone spur because he has had those before, and the pain is similar. Jerome also wears orthotics to compensate for his moderately flat feet **(pes planus).** A therapist and sports medicine physician assess his feet and lower extremities and notice that the feet are pronated, the Achilles' tendons are tight with limited dorsiflexion, and the

R leg is a bit longer than the **L.** Palpation reveals that the medial and middle plantar surface is a bit tender to the touch. The therapist evaluated the **Big Toe Sign** (first **MTP** pressed into extension), and it is positive for pain.

Identification of the Anatomy

The foot and ankle are complicated dissections, and tissue must be delicately isolated to reap the full benefit of identifying appropriate structures.

Appreciate the following structures during dissection:

For the purpose of this case, focus on the following structures once you have completed the full dissection in this exploration:

> Talocrural, subtalar, and mid tarsal joints
> The stirrup muscles of the ankle and foot
> Calcaneus, talus, navicular, and cuneiforms
> Tarsal sinus and calcaneal tuberosity
> Anterior talofibular ligament, deltoid ligament, and anterior-inferior tibiofibular ligament

Spring ligament, long and short plantar ligaments
Achilles' (calcaneal) tendon
Respective retinaculae
Tibialis anterior muscle
Plantar aponeurosis and deeper layers of muscle groupings

Questions

1. Given your understanding of the way we stress soft tissue, especially in weight-bearing structures, what structure of the foot may be the culprit of the pain?
2. Can you identify what brought on or predisposed Jerome to this injury?
3. What does the big toe sign stretch?

Discussion

Although Jerome was an avid tennis player and a good recreational athlete, he failed to realize that running is a different sport requiring different muscle strength and endurance. His overly zealous approach to training has had a deleterious effect on his training schedule. The condition he has is called **plantar fasciitis (PF)**, which stems from overuse and excessive training of his pes planus, and possibly the tight heel cords as well. PF is an acute inflammation of the medial border of the plantar fascia (or aponeurosis), causing pain whenever the foot is loaded. Jerome's early morning pain is the result of the change from planterflexed position of the foot during sleep to dorsiflexed position when he stands up. This transition stretches the structures that are tight, and pain is therefore immediate. Heel spurs **(osteophytes)** are also common in the foot but generally occur as osteophytic changes on the anterior calcaneal tuberosity or at the posterior surface of the calcaneus. The spurs are very tender and can be seen on a radiograph. The big toe sign provokes big extension and stretches the fascia connected to the first **MTP** when they are fully weight bearing. Unfortunately, PF is not an easy condition to treat, and interventions built on stretching, strengthening of associated musculature, and use of orthotics and modalities such as iontophoresis and preventative activities have shown to be helpful. In some instances, a surgical partial release of the aponeurosis may be indicated. As a rehabilitation professional, you can address and *fix* many things in patients, but correcting poor judgment is much more difficult.

Preparation

Refer to the articulated skeleton, and review the bony anatomy of the distal tibiofibula (N513, 514; G5.53, 5.59; GY309; C446, 447).
Identify:

Tibial (medial) malleolus
Groove for the tibialis posterior and flexor digitorum longus tendons
Fibular (lateral) malleolus
Malleolar fossa

Refer to the articulated foot skeleton (N523, 524; G5.56, 5.58, 5.67; GY310, 311; C450, 451).
Identify:

Talus
Navicular
Calcaneus
Cuboid
Cuneiforms (medial, intermediate, and lateral)
Metatarsals
Phalanges

Note that the tarsals, when packed together, form medial and longitudinal arches bound by deep plantar ligaments (N527, 528; G5.86; GY331, 332; C450, 455) (Figure 21-1). Especially, note the **plantar calcaneonavicular ligament,** or **spring ligament,** and the **long** and **short plantar ligaments.**

On a flexible articulated skeleton of the foot, examine the relationships of the talocrural joint, subtalar joint, and the transverse tarsal (midtarsal) joint.

TALOCRURAL JOINT

The axis of rotation for the talocrural joint runs transversely through the medial and lateral malleoli but slightly obliquely, with the medial pole more distal (Figure 21-2). Hence plantarflexion has a slight inversion component, directing the sole medially. Dorsiflexion has an eversion component, directing the sole somewhat laterally. The talocrural joint capsule is reinforced by the medial and lateral collateral ligaments (N527; G5.73, 5.75; GY316, 317; C452, 453). The **lateral collateral ligament** has three components: the **anterior** and **posterior talofibular ligaments**

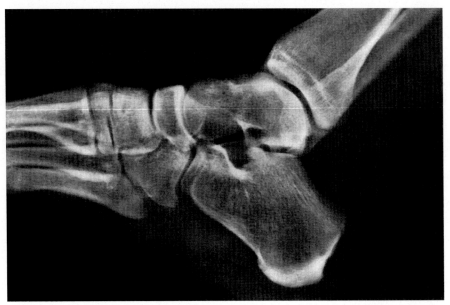

FIGURE 21-1
Mediolateral radiograph of the tarsals. *(From Wicke L:* Atlas of radiologic anatomy, *ed 7, Munich, 2001, Urban & Fischer.)*

and the **calcaneofibular ligament.** These ligaments are involved in common inversion sprains. The **medial collateral ligament,** or **deltoid ligament,** has four components: the **anterior** and **posterior tibiotalar ligaments** and the **tibionavicular** and **tibiocalcaneal ligaments.** These ligaments are involved in the less-common eversion sprains.

To expose the deltoid ligament, open the sheaths surrounding the tendons of the tibialis anterior and tibialis posterior, and retract them. Then, remove the synovium and connective tissue adherent to the underlying fibers of the ligament. Confirm its attachments to the talus and the navicular and sustentaculum tali of the calcaneus.

SUBTALAR JOINT

The axis of rotation for the subtalar joint passes obliquely through the calcaneal tuberosity and the talar head. This joint can be visualized as a mitered joint between the leg and the foot. Medial rotation of the leg in weight bearing imposes pronation of the foot (a combination of calcaneal eversion and talar plantarflexion). Lateral rotation of the leg in weight bearing imposes supination of the foot (calcaneal inversion and talar dorsiflexion). The principle ligament uniting the calcaneus and talus is the **interosseus talocalcaneal ligament,** which is found within the **tarsal sinus** (N527; G5.75; GY316; C452).

TRANSVERSE TARSAL (MID TARSAL) JOINT

The transverse tarsal joint is a compound joint composed of the talonavicular and the calcaneocuboid joints. The axis of rotation of the transverse tarsal joint is roughly longitudinal but inclined distally and deviated medially. The transverse tarsal joint permits the forefoot to remain evenly on the ground during supination and pronation of the hindfoot. When the hindfoot is pronated the joints of the transverse tarsal joint are loose-packed and mobile, capable of compensatory changes to conform to the ground. When the hindfoot is supinated the joints are close packed and stable elements of the longitudinal arch, which occurs when the foot functions as a rigid lever during the latter half of the stance phase of gait. The arch is supported in part by the **plantar calcaneonavicular (spring) ligament** and the **long plantar ligament** and **plantar calcaneocuboid ligament (short plantar ligament)** (N527, 528; G5.86; GY331, 332; C450, 455). Reflect the sectioned quadratus plantae and the tendon of the flexor digitorum longus to reveal these ligaments.

Anatomic Overview

The hallmark of the primate foot is the enlarged divergent great toe, or **hallux,** that permits the foot to grasp in a similar fashion to a hand. The

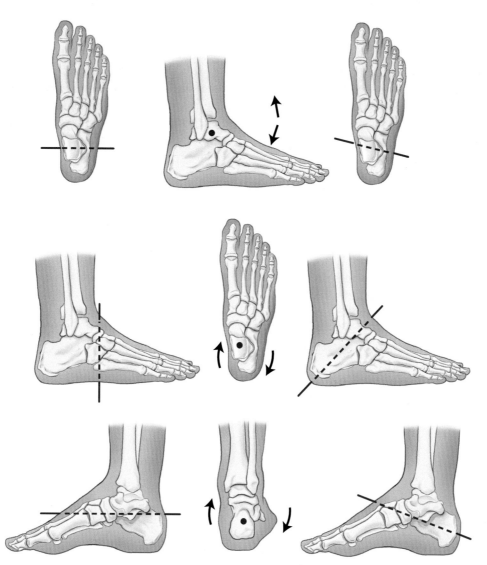

FIGURE 21-2

Axes of rotation of the talocrural, subtalar, and transverse tarsal joints. The first column indicates the generalized orientation of the axes; the second column indicates the rotation of the foot about the axes; the third column depicts a more lifelike orientation of the axes.

human foot is distinct in the loss of the divergence of the hallux, although any aspects of the musculoskeletal anatomy of the human foot reflect this prehensile legacy. Take particular note of the compromises between the function of the foot as a stable platform on which to stand and the retention of sufficient mobility to permit accommodation of the irregular surfaces encountered when walking, running, and climbing bipedally.

As you prepare to dissect, refer to the distribution of cutaneous innervation over the plantar foot (N541; G5.5; GY347; C366, 367). Trace the **saphenous nerve, sural nerve,** and **superficial peroneal nerve** into the foot. *What is the source of the sural nerve?* The sole of the foot is supplied by branches of the tibial nerve, that is, the **medial calcaneal branches** and the **medial** and **lateral plantar nerves** (S2-S3). Also review the superficial venous drainage (N544, 545; G5.10; GY344; C398, 412, 406). Generally, the posterolateral portions of the foot drain into the **lesser saphenous vein,** whereas the anteromedial portions flow into the **great saphenous vein.**

Dissection

Turn the cadaver into a prone position. **Note** the thick skin on the plantar aspect of the foot. The skin is devoid of hair follicles and covered with friction ridges or dermatoglyphics. The layer of lifeless keratinized cells, the **stratum corneum,** can be exceptionally thick here.

The underlying superficial fascia is compartmentalized by complex connective tissue septa and trabeculae that serve to anchor the skin and fascia firmly to the **plantar aponeurosis (N532; G5.66; GY336; C422).** The plantar aponeurosis arises from the **calcaneal tuberosity,** and its distal fibers divide to insert on both sides of the flexor tendons (Figure 21-3). Some fibers reach the bases of the proximal phalanges. When the toes are dorsiflexed, as in the latter half of the stance phase of gait, the plantar aponeurosis is made taut by the windlass mechanism (a **windlass** is a device for hauling or lifting, consisting of a drum on which the rope winds, and is turned by means of a crank),

thus lending support to the longitudinal arch of the foot. Attempt to dorsiflex the toes of the cadaver, and feel the tension in the plantar aponeurosis.

The margins of the aponeurosis have vertical septa that divide the plantar foot into three compartments: medial, intermediate, and lateral. Note that the medial and lateral plantar fascias are not as thick as the plantar aponeurosis.

The structures of the foot are typically considered as a series of layers. Once past the plantar aponeurosis, four layers generally remain.

FIRST LAYER
(N533; G5.67; GY337; C342)

Cut the plantar aponeurosis longitudinally down its center, then **make** two transverse cuts at either end, which reveals the **flexor digitorum brevis.**

Clean away the medial plantar fascia to reveal the **abductor hallucis.**

Clean away the lateral plantar fascia to expose the **abductor digiti minimi.**

Section all three of these muscles near their origins on the calcaneus, and **reflect** them distally.

SECOND LAYER
(N534; G5.68; GY338; C424)

Identify the tendons of the **flexor hallucis longus** and the **flexor digitorum longus.** The **quadratus plantae** (or flexor accessorius) is a short muscle that arises from the calcaneus and inserts on the obliquely oriented tendons of the flexor digitorum longus. Four **lumbricals** arise from the **flexor digitorum longus** tendons and insert on the medial aspects of the extensor expansions of the lateral four digits.

Cut the tendons of the **flexor hallucis longus** and **flexor digitorum longus** staggered, and **reflect** them distally.

TIP The tibial nerve on reaching the plantar compartment of the foot divides into two branches: the **medial plantar nerve (L4-L5) and lateral plantar** nerve (S1-S2). Their pattern of distribution is rather similar to that of the median and ulnar nerves in the hand; that is, the medial innervates the muscles associated with the hallux and the first lumbrical, *plus the flexor digitorum brevis,* and the lateral innervates all the remaining intrinsic muscles of the sole of the foot.

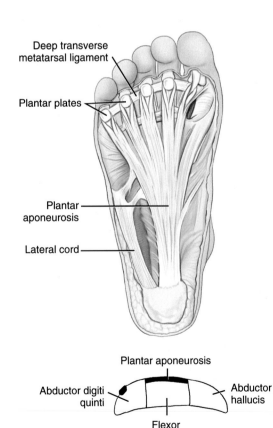

Deep transverse metatarsal ligament

Plantar plates

Plantar aponeurosis

Lateral cord

Plantar aponeurosis

Abductor digiti quinti

Abductor hallucis

Flexor digitorum brevis

FIGURE 21-3
Plantar aponeurosis.

THIRD LAYER

(N535; G5.69; GY339; C427)

Identify the **flexor hallucis brevis** with its medial and lateral head. The tendons contain two prominent sesamoid bones that lie beneath the head of the first metatarsal. The **adductor hallucis** has an oblique and a transverse head.

Locate the flexor digit minimi brevis.

Transect the oblique head of the adductor hallucis near its origin, and **reflect** it distally.

FOURTH LAYER

(N536, 53718; G5.70; GY340; C428)

The final layer consists of the **dorsal** and **plantar interossei.** The plantar interossei are unipennate and arise from the metatarsal of the digit onto which they insert. Just as in the hand, the plantar interossei adducts. Given that the functional axis of the foot lies about the second digit, the plantar interossei are found on digits three, four, and five.

The dorsal interossei are bipennate and arise from both metatarsals flanking the interosseus space. They abduct the toes and insert on digits two, three, and four.

TIP To help recall the actions of the plantar versus the dorsal interossei, think of the acronyms PAD and DAB. PAD indicates the Plantar interossei ADduct; DAB indicates the Dorsal ABduct the digits.

Although the muscles of the foot are anatomically dissected in four layers, functionally, they can be considered as being organized in three compartments: a medial compartment, containing the abductor hallucis and flexor hallucis brevis; a middle (or central) compartment, containing the flexor digitorum brevis, flexor digitorum longus, adductor hallucis, and lumbricals; and a lateral compartment, containing abductor digiti minimi and flexor digit minimi brevis (see Figure 21-3).

Exercises

1. In the figure below, color in and label each layer of the foot as seen in cross-section, and list its contents.

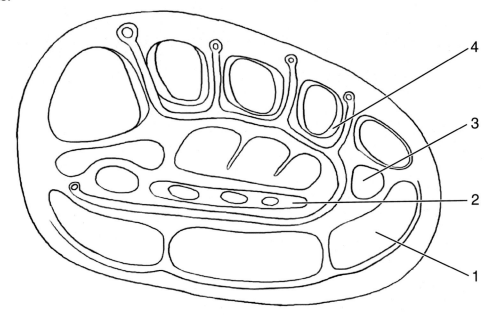

2. Heel pain is often associated with strains of the plantar aponeurosis. How do *heel spurs* relate to this type of pain?

3. The inversion sprain is the most common ankle injury. Explain why in terms of the range of motion at the ankle and the difference in size of the medial and lateral collateral ligaments.

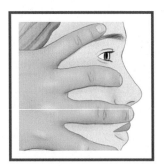

LAB EXPLORATION **22**

Viscerocranium and Muscles of Facial Expression

LAB OBJECTIVES

Dysfunction of the muscles of facial expression caused by palsy of the facial nerve can be a physically and psychologically debilitating condition. In this lab, you will examine the musculoskeletocutaneous basis of facial structure and its pattern of motor and sensory innervation. On completion of this lab, you should be able to:

- Describe the organization of the sensory innervation of the face and scalp.
- Identify the facial bones and designated landmarks.
- Summarize the derivation of facial muscles from the second branchial arch mesoderm.
- Identify the muscles of facial expression, and deduce their actions.

Preparation

Examine the disarticulated *(exploded)* and articulated skulls (N2, 4, 6; G7.2, 7.3; GY429-432; C514, 515, 530). Identify the often-delicate bones of the **facial skeleton.** Note the following landmarks:

   Piriform (nasal) aperture
   Orbital margin
   Supraorbital foramen
   Infraorbital foramen
   Mental foramen
   Nasolacrimal canal
   Stylomastoid foramen
   Zygomaticofacial foramen

Anatomic Overview

The bones of the facial skeleton form directly from sheets of undifferentiated **mesenchyme** aggregated within the dermis (Figure 22-1). Hence these bones

are called **intramembranous** or **dermal bones,** and they are formed by direct ossification. The mesenchyme cells become **osteoblasts** and begin to secrete **osteoid,** which gradually becomes mineralized, trapping the osteoblasts within the developing matrix of bones. Additional mesenchyme cells adjacent to this center of ossification differentiate into osteoblasts and enlarge it by appositional growth. The mesenchyme cells form an epithelial-like layer surrounding the bone, called the **periosteum.** Remodeling of the bone occurs as blood-borne monocytes become large multinucleated **osteoclasts,** which digest away the bony matrix. As the superficial surface of the bone grows through apposition, the deep surface is removed by the osteoclasts.

The **muscles of facial expression** are derived from the mesenchyme of the **second branchial arch** and are thus innervated by the cranial nerve **(CN)**

165

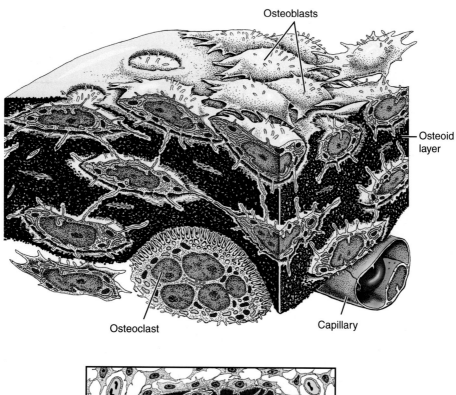

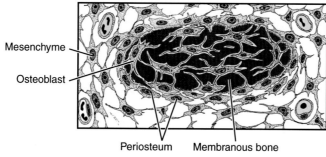

FIGURE 22-1

Structural histology of intramembranous or dermal bone. *(Modified from Krstic RV: General histology of the mammal, Berlin, 1984, Springer-Verlag.)*

associated with that arch, that is, the **facial nerve,** or **CN VII** (N123; G Table 9.9; GY458; C501). The muscles of facial expression are subcutaneous; that is, they lie within the superficial fascia. They attach from bone to skin, from skin to skin, or from deep fascia to skin. Therefore the superficial fascia must be left in place during the skinning procedure and the fat carefully and selectively cleaned away from the muscles afterward.

Cutaneous sensory innervation to the skin of the face and much of the anterior scalp is supplied by the nerve of the **first branchial arch,** the **trigeminal nerve,** or **CN V** (N122; G Table 9.5; GY455; C476). Additional sensory innervation is supplied by the dorsal and ventral rami of cervical spinal nerves 2 and 3 (N24; G Table 7.2; C499).

Dissection

Incise the skin shallowly over the face in the midline from bregma to the **mentum** (most prominent point on the chin) (Figure 22-2).

Make circular incisions about the orbital margin, the lower half of the nose, and the labial margins.

Carefully reflect the skin, leaving the superficial fascia in place. **Begin** at the corners formed by the intersection of your incisions in the lower portions of the face. The facial skin is very thin.

> **TIP** The skin over the forehead and scalp will be tightly adhered to the underlying deep fascia. If the scalp comes away easily, you are in the areolar space beneath the **galea aponeurotica** or **epicranial aponeurosis.**

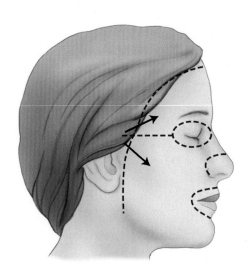 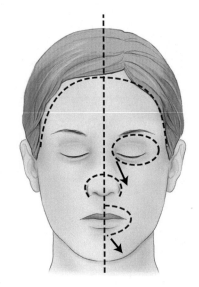

FIGURE 22-2
Skin incisions on the face.

Carefully clean and **identify** the facial muscles, noting their attachments, and **observe** their fiber orientations. These muscles are thin and delicate, especially in geriatric cadavers, and lie within the superficial fascia

TIP Using a new scalpel blade, clean away the obscuring fascia, and reveal the muscle fascicles. The backside of the tip of the scalpel dragged along the fascicles can help distinguish their fiber orientation. Clean and delineate the margins of the muscles, especially where they overlap. In many instances, their boundaries are indicated by an abrupt change in fiber orientation.

The contrast in texture and appearance between the muscle tissue and surrounding adipose tissue will become evident.

Identify the following, and, based on their points of attachment, **surmise** their actions (N26; G7.12, 7.15; GY456, 457; C494, 495):

Frontalis
Corrugator
Procerus
Orbicularis oculi
Nasalis
Zygomaticus major (and minor, if differentiated)
Risorus
Levator anguli oris

Levator labii superioris
Levator labii superioris alequae nasi
Orbicularis oris
Buccinator
Depressor anguli oris
Depressor labii inferioris
Mentalis
Platysma

Note the **facial artery**, a branch of the **external carotid artery**, which winds its way over the inferior border of the mandible then follows a tortuous course to the corner of the mouth and on to the medial angle of the eye.

Expose the large **parotid salivary gland.** Glandular tissue has a distinctive appearance. Some researchers have compared it with the appearance of cauliflower. It is encased in a tough fascia.

Clean toward its anterior border, and attempt to **identify** branches of the facial nerve (CN VII) emerging from the anterior margin of the parotid gland (N25; G7.13; GY459; C495). The terminal branches of the facial nerve are loosely named based on their positions: **temporal, zygomatic, buccal, mandibular, and cervical** (Figure 22-3). **Follow** these branches to the muscles they innervate.

Review the branches of the trigeminal nerve, CN V (N122; G Table 9.5; GY455; C510).

Look for the cutaneous branches of the trigeminal nerve.

Identify the **supraorbital nerve** and **supratrochlear nerve** and branches of **ophthalmic division of the**

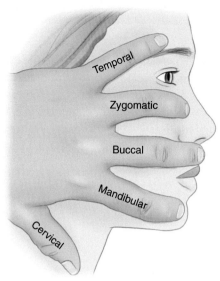

FIGURE 22-3
The branches of the facial nerve (CN VII).

trigeminal nerve (CN V^1) as they emerge near the supraorbital margin.

Cut the levator labii superioris near the infraorbital margin, and **reflect** the muscle belly caudally.

Identify the infraorbital nerve, a branch of the **maxillary division of the trigeminal nerve (CN V^2)**, where it emerges from the infraorbital foramen.

Using a clean fingertip, **tap** firmly on this spot on your own face, and **note** the tingling in your nose and upper lip.

Identify the **buccal** and **mental nerves,** branches of the **mandibular division of the trigeminal nerve (CN V^3).** The buccal nerve (not to be confused with the *buccal branches* of the facial nerve) passes medial to the masseter muscle.

Cut through the lower lip to the bone below the canine tooth on one side of the mouth. **Reflect** the corner of the cut posteriorly, and **cut** through the mucous membrane where it reflects from the gum to the lip, and **strip** the flap away from the bone, revealing the **mental nerve** emerging from the **mental foramen.**

Clinical Note

Bell's palsy

The most common disorder of the facial nerve is peripheral facial nerve paralysis, or Bell's palsy. This disorder involves all the muscles of facial expression (mimetic muscles) plus the **posterior belly of the digastric** and the **stylohyoid** muscles. The onset is sudden and may only last for a few hours and then disappear. Eighty percent of patients recover fully in a few weeks. The cause is usually some form of inflammation or compression of **CN VII** within the facial canal before it emerges from the **stylomastoid foramen.** Examine the accompanying illustration and discuss the muscles involved with the characteristic appearance of the palsy (Figure 22-4). *What additional functions may be compromised and what complications may ensue?*

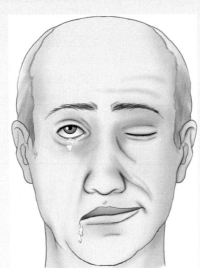

Paralyzed Side

Eye unable to close

No wrinkles

Tears pool

Facial muscles flabby and paralyzed

Corner of mouth lower

Drool

Normal Side

Eye voluntarily closed

Wrinkles present

Normal muscles pull face to normal side

FIGURE 22-4

The left side of the face exhibits symptoms of facial nerve palsy (Bell's palsy).

If the paralysis is complete, all of the muscles on one side of the face are affected. The affected side will appear smooth and wrinkleless because of the lack of muscle tone. For example, the furrows in the brow are missing because of the loss of tonus in the frontalis. The face will appear asymmetrical as a result of the unparalyzed side pulling on the flaccid side. The patient is unable to close the eye because of paralysis of the orbicularis occuli. Tears (lacrimation) may pool at the lateral corner of the eye, the palpebral fissure is extra wide, and the cornea is in danger of drying and ulceration. The nasolabial fold is lost because of paralysis of the zygomaticus major or minor (or both). The mouth cannot be closed properly because of loss of the orbicularis oris function. The affected corner hangs lower than normal, and saliva may drool from it. The patient cannot frown or grin because of paralysis of the depressor anguli oris and the risorius, respectively. Food accumulates between teeth and cheek because of paralysis of the buccinator.

In the case of an upper motor neuron lesion resulting from a cerebrovascular accident **(CVA)**, only the lower part of one side of the face would be affected. This circumstance occurs because the portion of the facial nucleus that innervates the upper quadrants of the face receives projections from both cerebral hemispheres. The patient would still be able to furrow the brow and close the eye on the side of the paralysis.

Exercises

1. Label the bones of the viscerocranium.

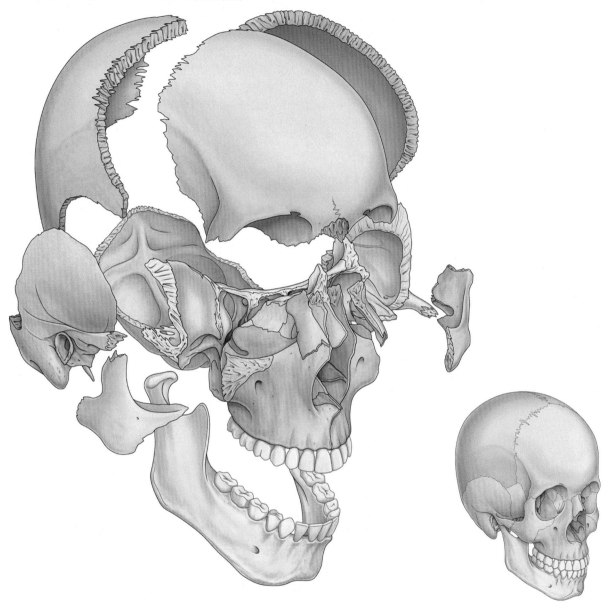

(From Drake R et al: *Gray's atlas of anatomy*, Philadelphia, 2008, Churchill Livingstone.)

2. On one side of the face, indicate the sensory fields of the three divisions of the trigeminal nerve (CN V). On the other side, indicate and label the points where the trigeminal nerve's principal cutaneous branches emerge from the skull.

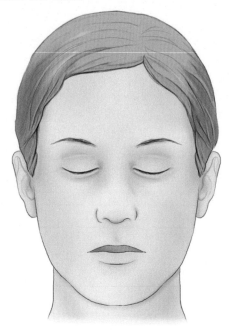

3. Draw in the peripheral course of the facial nerve (CN VII) once it emerges from the stylomastoid foramen, and indicate the five major groups of branches that supply motor innervation to the muscles of facial expression.

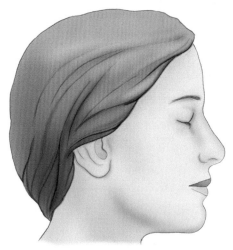

4. In facial nerve palsy, tears pool in the lateral corner of the eye. How do tears usually drain from the eye? How do the attachments, as well as subsequent paralysis of the orbicularis oculi, affect this situation?

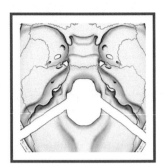

Neurocranium and Intracranial Fossae

LAB OBJECTIVES

In this lab, you will be exposing the neurocranium, removing the calvarium, and extracting the brain. This exercise will afford a consideration of the relationship of the brain and cranial nerves to the intracranial fossae and foramina. After completing this lab, you should be able to:

- Describe the layers of the scalp.
- Identify the bones of the neurocranium.
- Identify the meninges of the brain.
- Locate the cranial fossae, their foramina, and the neurovascular structures they transmit.
- Identify the cranial nerves on the brainstem.

Preparation

Refer to the articulated and exploded skull once again, and identify the bones of the **neurocranium** (N2, 4, 6; G7.2, 7.3; GY429-432; C514, 515, 530).

Identify the **suture joints** that unite these bones. *What type of joints are these (structurally and functionally)?* Examine a horizontally sectioned skull and the relative thickness of the bone at various points around its circumference. *Why might a blow to the temple pose particular risks?* Identify the following foramina and openings within the neurocranial fossae (N9, 11; G7.6; GY437; C531):

    Cribiform plate
    Optic canal
    Superior orbital fissure
    Foramen rotundum
    Foramen ovale
    Foramen spinosum
    Foramen lacerum
    Carotid canal

    Internal acoustic meatus
    Jugular foramen
    Hypoglossal canal

Keep the skull at your table to compare with the cadaver.

Anatomic Overview

Although much of your study of the brain will be deferred to a neuroscience course, this dissection affords you the opportunity to examine in situ the protective coverings of the brain, and you will better appreciate the topographic relationship of the brain and cranial nerves to the cranial base. As with the spinal nerves, the cranial nerves convey general sensory, general motor, and autonomic signals to and from structures of the head and other parts of the body. In addition, cranial nerves convey information from the special sensory organs concentrated in the head, such as those for vision, smell, hearing, balance, and taste.

The neurocranium is composed of the bones of the skull that lie in contact with the brain (Figure 23-1). Bones that form the vault of the cranium develop in similar fashion to those of the face—as dermal or intramembranous bones. Bones that form the cranial base, however, form indirectly by way of an intermediate cartilaginous model of the bone. This process is called **indirect** or **endochondral ossification.** In this case, the mesenchyme cells differentiate into **chondroblasts** that secrete an extracellular matrix of cartilage. It enlarges by **interstitial growth,** as chondroblasts within the matrix continue to secrete cartilage, and by appositional growth, as additional mesenchyme cells within the chondrogeneic layer of the **perichondrium** differentiate into chondroblasts around the periphery. In its early stages, the human cranial base looks remarkably similar to the chondrocranium of a shark.

Several centers of ossification appear as the cartilage begins to ossify. **Chondroclasts** begin to fill cavities within the calcified matrix, followed by newly differentiated osteoblasts, which begin to lay down osteoid. The process of ossification and

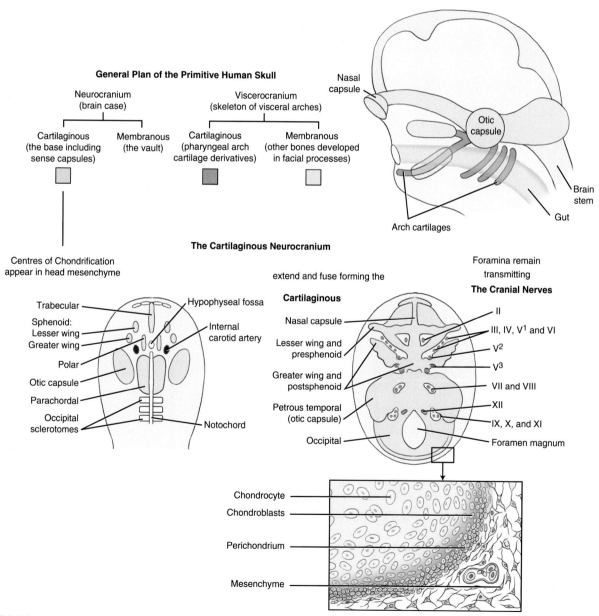

FIGURE 23-1

The relationships of neurocranium versus viscerocranium and membranous (direct) and cartilaginous (indirect) ossification.

remodeling proceeds. Thus endochondral ossification differs from intramembranous ossification by the intermediate step of a cartilaginous model of the bone. All of the remaining bones of the postcranial skeleton develop via endochondral ossification (except for portions of the clavicle) (Figure 23-2).

Dissection

Place the cadaver in a prone position with a block under the chest. At the cut edge of the scalp, **note** the sequential layers (N102; G7.16, 7.18; GY442; C520). They form the acronym SCALP:

Skin
Connective tissue
Aponeurosis (galea aponeurotica, or epicranialis)
Loose areolar connective tissue
Pericranium (periosteum)

Remove the remaining scalp. **Expose** the **temporalis fascia** (N54; G7.41; GY457; C498).

Reflect the temporalis muscle away from the parietal bone. **Note** the **superior** and **inferior temporal lines** (N4; G7.3; GY480; C515).

Place a large rubber band about the skull at approximately its widest points, or approximately 2 cm above the **supraorbital margin** and the **inion.**

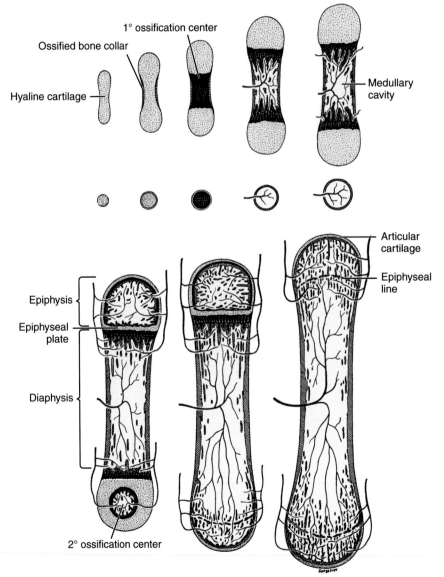

FIGURE 23-2
Endochondral (indirect) ossification in a long bone. (*Modified from Bloom W, Fawcett DW:* A textbook of Histology, *ed 9, IN, 1968, Saunders. Junqueira LC, Carneiro J, Contopoulos AN*: Basic histology, *ed 2, Los Altos, Calif, 1977, Lang Medical Publications.*)

With an oscillating saw, **carefully cut** the skull along the rubber band (Figure 23-3). Be careful, particularly on the sides of the calvarium where the bone is relatively thin, to avoid penetrating too deeply. **Refer** to a sectioned dry skull to gauge the depth better.

TIP As needed, complete the separation of the calvarium with a chisel and mallet. Pry the dura free with a blunt probe, an osteotome, or your fingers. *Be careful of sharp shards of bone that may remain around the skull rim.*

Review the muscles of the suboccipital region, and **carefully detach** those attached to the occipital bone (N178; G4.39; GY43; C440).

Remove a large wedge from the occipital bone by sawing a line from the lateral margin of the foramen magnum to the lambdoidal suture where it intersects the horizontal saw cut around the calvarium. **Repeat** on the opposite side. **Pry** the bone away from the dura mater.

Examine the dura mater (N99, 100; G7.18, 7.19; GY442; C521). **Note** the presence of the branches of the **middle meningeal artery,** the **superior sagittal sinus,** and the **arachnoid granulations.**

Incise the dura, and **detach** it from the **crista gali** (N103; G7.20; GY443; C522).

Incise the **tentorium cerebelli** along the margin of the petrosal bone and along the **transverse sinus.**

Section the spinal cord and vertebral arteries.

Gently lift the brain forward, and use a very sharp small scalpel to **section** the cranial nerves and

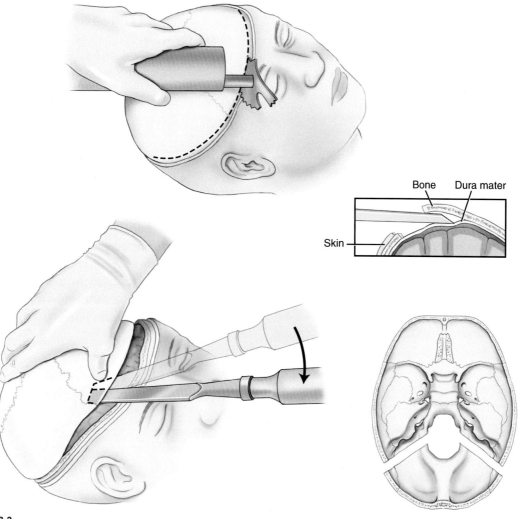

FIGURE 23-3
Exposure of the intracranial cavity.

internal carotid arteries as close to the bone as possible.

CRANIAL NERVES
(N118; G7.22, 7.23; GY451; C534)

Free the brain from the cranial cavity. **Rinse** and **examine** it, as time permits **(N105, 114; G7.84, 7.91; GY446; C426)**. Give particular attention to the cranial nerves seen on the ventral surface. Traditionally, the cranial nerves are designated by Roman numerals, ordered by the rostrocaudal emergence of the nerves from the ventral brainstem. A pneumonic is frequently cited to aid students in memorizing the order of the cranial nerves. It is a silly jingle that goes like this: "On old Olympus towering top a Finn and German viewed Austrian hops."

(Rostral)

On	I.	Olfactory
Old	II.	Optic
Olympus	III.	Oculomotor
Towering	IV.	Trochlear
Top	V.	Trigeminal
A	VI.	Abducens
Finn	VII.	Facial
And	VIII.	Acoustic (vestibulocochlear)
German	IX.	Glossopharyngeal
Viewed	X.	Vagus
Austrian	XI.	Accessory
Hops	XII.	Hypoglossal

(Caudal)

Rinse the interior of the cranial cavity, and **examine** the three **intracranial fossae: anterior, middle,** and **posterior.**

Use a sectioned dry skull as a reference **(N11; G7.6, 7.89; GY437; C531)**, and **identify** the cranial fossae and foramina and the structures they transmit **(N104; G7.22; GY450; C532)**. **Note** that some cranial nerves travel some distance beneath the dura before exiting the skull through a bony foramen.

Reflect the dura covering the trigeminal ganglion, and **trace** its three divisions.

Correlate the structures observed based on the brain with those in the cranial fossa.

Immerse and **store** the brain according to the directions of your instructor.

ARTERIES OF THE BRAIN
(N139-142; G7.28; CY454; C535)

Observe the two principal arterial supplies to the brain: the **internal carotid arteries** and the **vertebral arteries.** The internal carotid arteries enter the cranium via the **carotid canal**, loop through the **cavernous sinus**, then divide into two major branches. The smaller of these two branches is the **anterior cerebral artery.**

Trace the anterior cerebral artery forward into the **longitudinal cerebral fissure**, separating the two cerebral hemispheres where it follows the curve of the **corpus callosum.** The second and larger branch is the **middle cerebral artery. Follow** this artery in the **lateral sulcus** between the frontal and temporal lobes.

The vertebral arteries enter the cranium through the foramen magnum and unite to form the **basilar artery** lying on the ventral surface of the brainstem. Three paired branches supply the cerebellum: the **posterior inferior cerebellar artery, anterior inferior cerebellar artery,** and **superior cerebellar artery.** The basilar artery finally divides into the paired **posterior cerebral arteries.**

The carotid and the vertebral arterial circuits are united by anastomoses formed by the **anterior** and **posterior communicating branches,** creating the **cerebral arterial circle (circle of Willis).**

Exercises

1. Label the bones of the neurocranium.

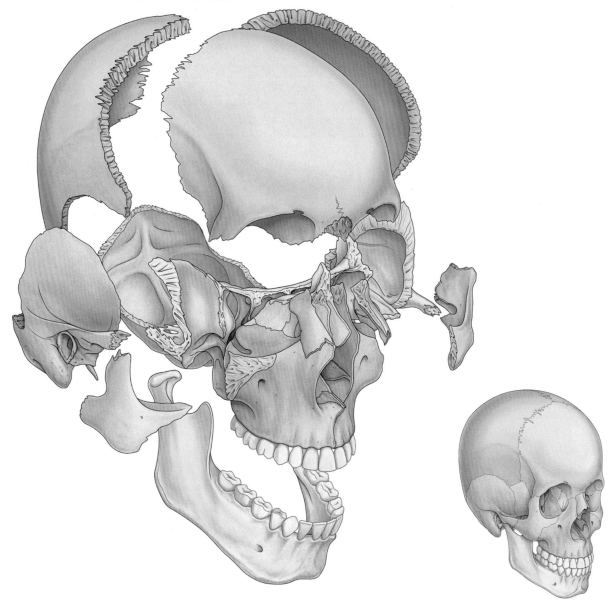

(From Drake R et al: *Gray's atlas of anatomy*, Philadelphia, 2008, Churchill Livingstone.)

2. Indicate the anterior, middle, and posterior cranial fossae. Label each foramen and indicate the structure transmitted.

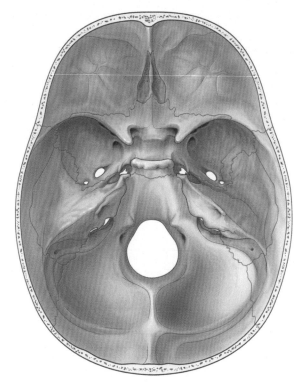

(From Drake R et al: *Gray's atlas of anatomy*, Philadelphia, 2008, Churchill Livingstone.)

3. Draw in the cranial nerves (except CN I) on the anterior view of the brainstem.

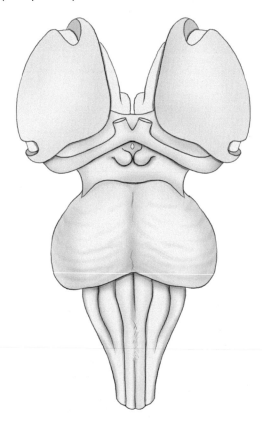

4. Locate and identify the following on the arteriogram:

cervical portion of internal carotid artery
petrous portion
cavernous portion (siphon) of internal carotid artery
anterior cerebral artery
middle cerebral artery

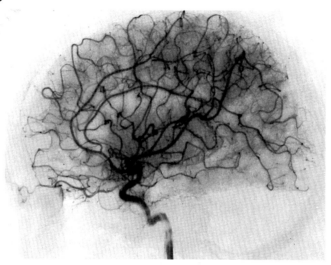

(From Adam, A and Adrian Dixon. *Grainger & Allison's Diagnostic Radiology 5e*, 2008, Churchill Livingstone.)

Muscles of Mastication and the Temporomandibular Joint

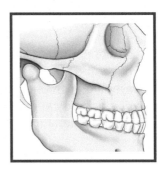

CASE STUDY

Temporomandibular Joint Disorder

An endodontist refers a 20 **y/o** patient to the physical medicine service for an evaluation of **R TMJ** pain and clicking after a gradual onset. The patient **c/o** pain and slight difficulty opening the mouth, which is accompanied by an audible *click*. She indicates that she noticed a slight **L** lateral deviation of the mandible when opening her mouth, with return to normal on closing, which was also accompanied by a *click*. She has full **AROM** of 45 mm of mandibular depression. Her pain is local at the **R TMJ** and sometimes radiates to the temporal region on the same side. She frequently experiences paresthesias in the external acoustic meatus. She also indicates that headaches occur some mornings. She wears a bite block to decrease the pressure during episodes of teeth grinding **(Bruxism)** during her sleep. Her upper quarter screen **(UQS)** is normal in all aspects.

Identification of the Anatomy

The temporomandibular joint complex (also known as the **TMJ**) is a unique structure because it serves an intricate function in guiding the depression, elevation, lateral excursion, retrusion, and protrusion of the mandible. A fibrous capsule is generally loose more medially than laterally and delineates the anatomic boundaries of the joint. Three accessory ligaments support the joint, which allow for the attachment of the cranium to the mandible. The joint has three degrees of freedom.

Appreciate the following structures during dissection:

Musculature
    Superficial:
        Masseter
        Temporalis
    Deep:
        Lateral pterygoid
        Medial pterygoid (and superior pterygoid)
        Digastric

Infrahyoid
Mylohyoid
Geniohyoid
Joint complex
Postglenoid spine
Mandibular fossa
Mandibular condyle
Articular eminence
Articular crest
Articular tubercle
Ligaments
Stylomandibular
Sphenomandibular
Temporomandibular
Soft tissue
Superior lamina
Disc-pars posterior
Inferior lamina
Upper and lower joint space
Auriculotemporal nerve
Masseteric nerve
Posterior deep temporal nerve

Questions

1. Given the signs, history, and symptoms of this case, what is the probable cause of the reciprocal click and pain in this patient?
2. What imbalance of muscle tension may be responsible for the mandibular deviation?
3. What is the cause of the paresthesia of the external acoustic meatus?

Discussion

Although the causes for pain, click, and deviation in the **TMJ** are numerous, this patient probably has a disc that is displaced anteriorly on the condyle in the resting position because of stretched superior and posterior disc attachments or possible capsular laxity caused by the chronic **Bruxism.** During mandibular depression, the mouth opens, and the condyle translates forward, riding over the displaced disc. As it slips into its proper position beneath the disc, it produces a clicking sound. The mandible then opens to full depression. When the mandible is fully elevated (mouth closing), the disc again slips anteriorly into the abnormal resting position, producing the reciprocal clicking sound. The mandibular deviation to the left may be caused by weakness in the **L** lateral and medial pterygoids, given that they function to track motion to the opposite side. The auriculotemporal nerve passes just posterior to the **TMJ.** Inflammation of the joint may

irritate the nerve, causing paresthesia in areas supplied with sensory innervation by its branches, including the skin lining the external acoustic meatus. The **TMJ** undergoes many changes to cause temporomandibular joint disorder **(TMJD).** Trauma, faulty dentition, abnormality in condylar surfaces, arthritis, acromegalia, and tumors can affect this joint. Keep in mind: an audible click or crepitus on opening and closing may be normal in an otherwise functional joint.

Preparation

Identify on the **skull** (N4, 10, 14; G7.3, 7.5, GY432, 436; C515):
Superior and inferior temporal lines
Zygomatic arch
Mastoid process
Mandibular fossa
External acoustic meatus
Styloid process
Pterygoid process
Identify on the **mandible** (N15; G7.40; GY479; C504, 505):
Condylar process
Coronoid process
Ramus: angle and body
Lingula
Pterygoid fossa

Anatomic Overview

Cells from the **fourth somitomere** migrate into the **first branchial arch** to become the muscle cells associated with the skeletal elements derived from this arch. The trigeminal somitomere gives rise to nine muscles, six of which act to move the mandible during chewing. These muscles are the **temporalis, masseter, superior pterygoid, medial pterygoid, lateral pterygoid,** and **anterior belly of the digastric muscles.** They are innervated by motor branches of the trigeminal nerve (cranial nerve [CN] V). The maxilla and mandible are dermal bones that replace the first branchial arch cartilages (**Meckel's cartilage** and the **palatopterygoquadrate**).

Dissection

Review your dissection of the parotid region and the structures radiating from the anterior border of the parotid gland (N23, 25; G7.12, 7.13; GY458; C500).

Use blunt dissection as much as possible, and **remove** the parotid gland from its fascial bed, tracing the branches of the **facial nerve** (CN VII) back toward the **stylomastoid foramen (N10, 123; G7.5, G Table 9.9; GY436; C513).**

TIP The parotid gland is invested by a tough fascia that makes removing it by blunt dissection a challenge. First, identify a branch of the facial nerve emerging from its anterior border, and then, using a scissor technique, trace the nerve centrally through the gland toward the stylomastoid foramen. Accomplishing this task for one or two branches will be sufficient.

Follow the temporal branches of the facial nerve until you locate the **auriculotemporal nerve** (a branch of CN V³) lying just anterior to the external ear **(N24, 122; G7.13, 7.42, 7.47, G Table 9.5; GY455; C512).**
Trace the auriculotemporal nerve toward the neck of the mandible. Irritation of this nerve in TMJD may cause paresthesia over its area of cutaneous distribution.
Clean the **masseter,** and **detach** the posterior (deep) portion of the muscle from the zygomatic arch.
Reflect the masseter forward to reveal the **masseteric nerve** passing through the **mandibular notch (N54; G7.41, C512).**
Saw through the zygomatic arch just anterior to the TMJ, and **make** a second cut as far forward as possible **(N55; G7.41; GY480)** (Figure 24-1).
Reflect the arch with its attached masseter muscle inferiorly. **Note** that the deep fibers attach to the superior portion of the **mandibular ramus** and the lateral surface of the **coronoid process (N54; G7.41; GY480; C499). Leave** the superficial fibers attached to the inferior margin of the mandible.
Cut through the coronoid process of the mandible with a saw, **reflect** it with the attached **temporalis muscle,** and **pin** it back.
Locate the **lingula** on the medial surface of the dry mandible, and **estimate** its position on the cadaver mandible.
Slide a blunt probe under the ramus and down against the lingula.
Use the bone saw to make a series of shallow parallel cuts through the lateral cortical layer of bone just below the estimated position of the lingula.
Use an osteotome to remove carefully the cortical bone, and **expose** the **inferior alveolar nerve** in its canal. When the nerve is located, **cut** the ramus of the mandible at the level of the **mandibular foramen,** sparing the inferior alveolar nerve.

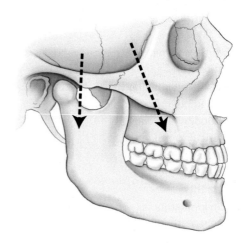

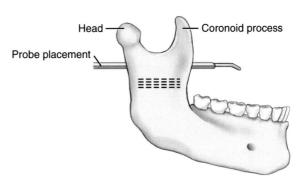

FIGURE 24-1
Removal of the zygomatic arch and exposure of the inferior alveolar nerve.

Cut the **mandibular neck,** and **remove** the detached piece of bone.
Examine the **infratemporal fossa. Observe** the maxillary artery, a branch of the external carotid artery, arising posterior to the neck of the mandible. **Identify** the **inferior alveolar nerve, lingual nerve, mylohyoid nerve,** and branches of CN V³ **(N46, 71; G7.42; GY483; C513).**
Clean the **medial** and **lateral pterygoid muscles (N55; G7.42; GY480; C502, 503).**

The lateral pterygoid muscle has two heads. The superior head is considered by some researchers to be a separate muscle, the **superior pterygoid.** It arises from the roof of the fossa and inserts on the front of the TMJ capsule and the **articular disc (N55; G7.45, 7.46; GY481, 482).** The inferior head of the lateral pterygoid arises from the lateral surface of the **lateral pterygoid plate** of the sphenoid bone and attaches on the neck of the mandible. The medial pterygoid arises from the medial surface of the lateral pterygoid plate, and the **maxillary tuberosity** then inserts on the medial surface of the mandibular ramus (N55; G7.42; GY480).

Identify these points of attachment on a dry skull.

TEMPOROMANDIBULAR JOINT

Note the lateral thickening of the joint capsule forming the **temporomandibular ligament** (N16; G7.45). The anterior portion of the capsule is thin and loose, which, when combined with the incongruence of the joint surfaces, predisposes the joint to anterior dislocation. **Verify** the two movements possible at this joint: hinge and protraction or retraction. To further appreciate these movements, **place** your little finger in your own external ear canal, and **feel** the **mandibular condyle** as you open or close and protract or retract your jaw.

Open the joint capsule, and **observe** the articular disc (N16, 55; G7.46; GY481; C502). **Note** the attachments of the superior pterygoid muscle. The disk divides the TMJ into two separate joint spaces, each with its own synovium. The lower joint is a hinge joint. **Determine** the axis of rotation. The upper joint is a gliding joint. *How does this movement influence the functional position of the axis of rotation of the mandible during mastication?*

Exercises

1. Draw in the fibers of the medial and lateral pterygoid muscles.

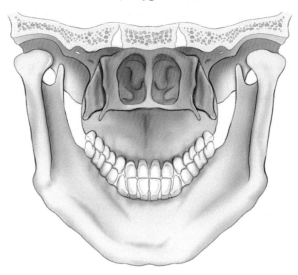

2. Indicate on the mandible the axis of rotation during mastication. What anatomic landmarks are coincident with this point? What is the significance of this position of the axis of rotation for the inferior alveolar nerve?

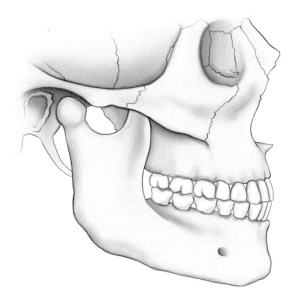

3. In one person, the audible click accompanying depression of the jaw is heard almost instantly. In the second, it occurs later. What is the significance of the timing of the click for dysfunction of the TMJ?

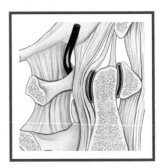

LAB EXPLORATION 25

Craniovertebral Joints and Prevertebral Muscles

LAB OBJECTIVES

In this lab, we will separate the head from the vertebral column so as to explore the ligaments of the atlantooccipital and atlantoaxial joints and to examine the prevertebral musculature. On completion of this lab, the student should be able to:

- Distinguish the specialized features of the atlas (C1) and the axis (C2).
- Describe the anatomy and function of the atlantooccipital and atlantoaxial joints.
- Describe the compartmentalization of the neck.
- Name the attachments, actions, and innervations of the prevertebral muscles.
- Discuss the basis of *whiplash* strains of the prevertebral muscles.

CASE STUDY

The Office Headache

Christa is a 52 **y/o** accountant for the National Engineering Laboratory and was recently transferred to the accounting department from external grant auditing. Christa has been in this position for 2 weeks and visits the on-site occupational medicine department with neck stiffness and a worrisome **HA** that seems to worsen during the day and, at times, becomes so bad that she needs to lie down to alleviate the symptoms. Her social history indicates that she did not have this issue in the grants department and has noticed the **HA** gradually over the last week. She hints that her new supervisor can be "difficult," and perhaps the pain is just the stress of new expectations in this new branch of the corporation. She suggests that moving out of her desk position also helps

the symptoms. Her **PMH** is negative for neck trauma or any **TMJD.** She also offers that her sister has had terrible migraine headaches and hopes this episode is not the start of similar problems. Christa denies any problems with vision, hearing, or swallowing. She points to the area of the occipital region and the lateral and posterior sides of the neck as being the most painful.

Identification of the Anatomy

The dissection in this Exploration involves identifying the deeper components of the craniovertebral and prevertebral structures; these components are intricately involved with the posterior, anterior, and superficial muscular and ligamentous components of the same region. As noted in several instances in this text, the movements of the C1 and C2 vertebrae are essential in the overall movement of the head, and numerous ligaments, muscles, and joints help orchestrate both the stability and the mobility of the head and neck in daily function. Take time to review the muscles of the suboccipital triangle in Exploration Lab 3 and the neck triangles in Exploration Lab 10.

Appreciate the following structures during dissection:

Anterior and posterior longitudinal ligaments
Prevertebral fascia
Posterior arch
Dens
Transverse ligament of the atlas
Alar ligament
Apical ligament
Cruciform ligament
Posterior atlantooccipital ligament
Occipital condyles
Muscles of the occipital triangle
Suboccipital nerve
Scalene triangle musculature and its borders
Sternocleidomastoid muscles
Upper trapezius
Semispinalis cervicis and capitis

Questions

1. What anterior, posterior, and lateral structure would be stretched and shortened in positions of full extension, flexion, and lateral rotation?
2. From the case description, what factors can you identify that may be directly or indirectly related to the cause of the **HA** and neck pain.
3. What are the differences between the presentations of *tension* compared with migraine headaches?

Discussion

Christa has several issues that may be causing her stiffness and **HA.** As health care providers, we need to conduct a thorough history with the patient to ascertain and to rule out causative factors for the related signs and symptoms of a patient compliant. In this case, a very critical component may be related to the patient's current workstation because it is different than her previous one. She hints at this factor when she suggests that the symptoms improve when she moves away from the desk and that signs and symptoms get worse as she continues to work. If the neck is positioned in poor posture, then structures are likely to be stretched or shortened. Forward head posture, for example, places the sternocleidomastoid **(SCM)**

muscle on stretch and the suboccipital muscles on tension. This circumstance may cause muscle spasm or co-contraction on movement, which may elicit some of the symptoms in this case or initiate *trigger points* in the muscles that refer pain elsewhere. This patient most likely has a *tension-type* **HA** defined as a headache with a feeling of tightness, constriction, or pressure that widely vary in frequency and intensity but are long lasting and are usually related to muscular tension and life stress. The classifications of **HA** are many and complicated, but the symptoms in this case do not suggest a migraine. Many types of **HA** exist—from tension to *cluster*—but migraines (neuropathic or vascular) have been shown to elicit some classic signs and symptoms, including a prodromal event, episodes lasting at least 4 hours and occurring at least two times, unilateral hemispherical throbbing pain (commonly retroorbital, photophobic, or phonophobic), and nausea with or without vomiting. Christa does have some family history that may be applicable to migraine, but the vast majority of her symptoms are not indicative of this major health problem.

Preparation

Identify the bony landmarks of the cervical spine and cranial base (N10, 17; G4.11, 4.12, 7.5; GY24, 436; C342, 536):

Atlas (all parts)
Axis (all parts)
Occipital condyles
Foramen magnum
Dorsum sella
Clivus
Basioccipital
Basisphenoid

Anatomic Overview

Examine a figure or model of the head and neck in sagittal section and cross-section (N35, 63; G8.1; GY490; C587). The **investing fascia** is continuous with the deep fascia over the sternocleidomastoid and trapezius muscles. It completely surrounds, or invests the neck.

Within the neck are two compartments. The anterior compartment is called the **visceral compartment** and contains the **trachea, esophagus, carotid arteries, internal jugular veins,** and **vagus nerves.** It is partitioned by a series of connective tissue layers. The **pretracheal fascia** and the **buccopharyngeal fascia** surround the trachea and esophagus and are fused to the **carotid sheaths,** which enclose the carotid artery, jugular vein, and vagus nerve on either side. The posterior compartment is called the **vertebral compartment.** It is encompassed by the **prevertebral fascia,** which surrounds the vertebral column, epaxial muscles, and prevertebral muscles (Figure 25-1).

The visceral and vertebral compartments are readily separated at the **retrovisceral (retropharyngeal) space,** a potential space containing loose connective tissue extending from the base of the skull into the upper mediastinum of the thorax.

Dissection

Cut the **posterior atlantooccipital membrane** (N21; G4.13; C343).

Use bone snips to **remove** the **posterior arch** of the atlas.

Turn to the posterior cranial fossa, and **incise** the dura mater on the basisphenoid just below the **dorsum sella. Use** a blunt instrument such as a spatulate probe to **reflect** it inferiorly and to expose the **tectorial membrane** (N22; G4.14; GY489) (Figure 25-2).

Clinical Note

Whiplash—hyperextension

The abrupt lurch forward accompanying a rear-end motor-vehicle collision frequently results in a *whiplash* injury to the neck. Hypertension of the cervical region of the vertebral column may result in strains or tears of structures disposed to resist this type of movement, namely, the anterior longitudinal ligament and the prevertebral muscles. An abrupt stop by the vehicle may also produce a hyperflexion injury in a person restrained by a seatbelt as the head snaps forward onto the chest, which may result in injury to the structures that resist this movement, namely the posterior longitudinal ligament, ligamentum flavum, supraspinous ligament, and the extensor muscles of the neck. In addition, excessive compression of the cervical intervertebral discs may result in tears of the annulus fibrosus and protrusion of the nucleus pulposus, especially in older individuals in whom the disc water content is diminished.

Note that the tectorial membrane is continuous with the **posterior longitudinal ligament** (Figure 25-3).

Cut the tectorial membrane just above the anterior border of the foramen magnum, and **reflect** it inferiorly to expose the deeper ligaments. **Proceed**

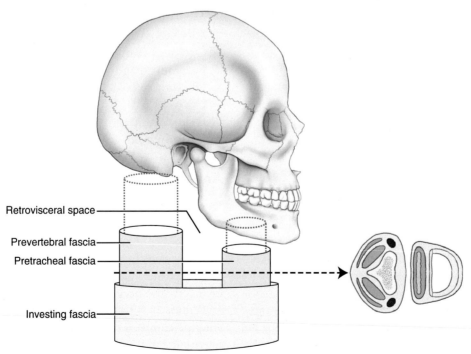

FIGURE 25-1
Vertebral and visceral compartments of the neck.

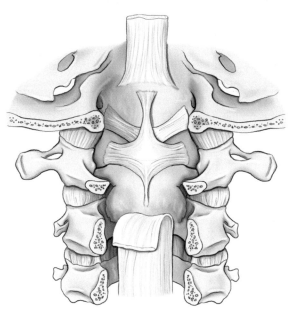

FIGURE 25-2
Reflection of the tectorial membrane to expose the cruciate and alar ligaments.

carefully because the tectorial membrane may be adherent to the **superior longitudinal band.** It can be more readily distinguished from the **transverse ligament of the atlas** because the fibers run perpendicular to those of the tectorial membrane.

The **dens** of the axis is held in place by the **transverse ligament,** which, together with the superior and inferior bands, constitute the **cruciform ligament.** The cruciform (cruciate) ligament holds the dens in place and allows the skull and atlas to rotate as a unit on the axis.

Spanning from the dens to the occipital bone are the **alar ligaments,** or **check ligaments.** These ligaments can be nearly the diameter of a pencil in girth. They check the lateral rotation of the head.

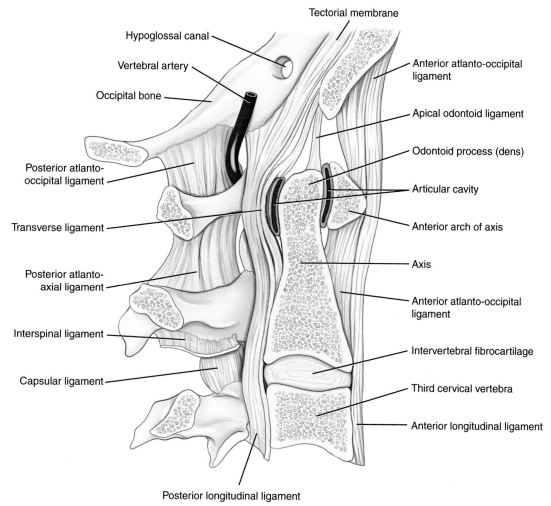

FIGURE 25-3
Sagittal section through the cranial vertebral joints and ligaments.

Observe the extent of lateral rotation possible in the cadaver. Now, **cut** the alar ligaments close to the dens, and **repeat** the movement.

Cut the superior band of the cruciform ligament and the deeper **apical ligament** of the dens.

Cut through the joint capsules along the medial and posterior sides of the **occipital condyles** opening the **atlantooccipital joints.**

Force a chisel into the joints, and **force** them open as much as possible.

TIP Turn the cadaver over into a supine (face-up) position. Before continuing, be sure your dissection of the posterior triangle of the neck (**N28; G8.5; C480**) is complete, and review the course of the spinal accessory nerve and branches of the cervical plexus. Clean the surfaces of the **anterior, middle,** and **posterior scalene** muscles and the **levator scapulae.** Review their attachments (**N26; G Table 8.6, 8.7; C488**).

Place your hands into the **retrovisceral space,** and **pull** the cervical fascia forward (**N35, 63; G8.1; GY490; C587**).

Move your hands upward, and **feel** the prominent transverse process of the atlas (**N30; G Table 8.4; GY493; C488**).

Sever the **rectus capitis lateralis** and the **rectus capitis anterior** on each side. These muscles span between the transverse process of the atlas and the occipital bone.

Sever the thick **longus capitis** running between the anterior tubercles of C3 through C6 and the occipital bone.

Pass your scalpel between the skull and atlas, and **cut** the **anterior atlantooccipital membrane,** which is continuous with the **anterior longitudinal ligament** (**N21; G4.13; C343**).

Reflect the head and visceral compartment forward and downward to expose the prevertebral and lateral vertebral (scalene) muscles. **Examine** the deep fascia over these muscles. This **prevertebral fascia** is often bilaminar over the vertebral bodies. The most anterior layer is called the **alar fascia** (**N35, 63; G8.1; GY490; C587**). Attempt to **separate** these layers, and then **clean** and **identify** the **longus colli, longus capitis, scalenes,** and **levator scapulae** muscles.

Exercises

1. Match the following structures in the neck to their homologs in the thoracic vertebral column.

    ____ Tectorial membrane
    ____ Ligamentum nuchae
    ____ Posterior atlantooccipital membrane
    ____ Anterior atlantooccipital membrane

    a. Ligamentum flavum
    b. Anterior longitudinal ligament
    c. Supraspinous ligament
    d. Posterior longitudinal ligament

2. Draw in the prevertebral muscles on the accompanying diagram.

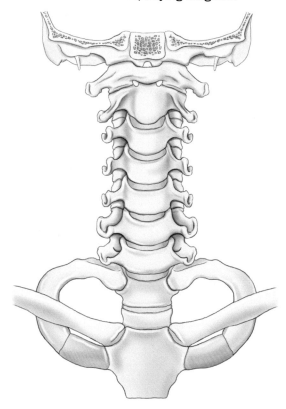

3. Draw in and name a structure that prevents the dens from crushing the spinal cord and a structure that prevents excessive rotation of the skull about the axis.

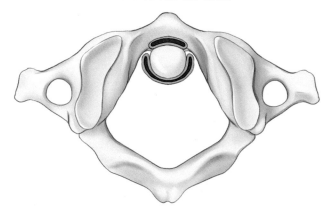

4. What is the functional reason for the absence of an intervertebral disc between C1 and C2?

5. About what axis of rotation does extension of the neck occur?

Index

Printed in the United States
By Bookmasters